THE WELL BOOKS

thewellbooks@gmail.com

© STUART DEEKS 2009

Stuart Deeks asserts the moral right to be
identified as the author of this work.

A catalogue record of this book is
available from the British Library.

ISBN 978-0-9564472-0-3
Published by The Well Books
First Edition : December 2009

Book Design by John Jolly

Cover Illustration by Solveig Oliver
Back Cover: Drawing by 11 year old girl
after benefit from Plastic wrap, the remedy.

This book is printed with soya based inks on stocks from
well-managed forests and other controlled sources by
Cambrian Printers Ltd,
Llanbadarn Road, Aberystwyth, SY23 3TN
www.cambrian-printers.co.uk

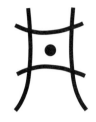

The Well

A common source of strength that all can rely on.

It is a structure that allows access to the source – one finds
what supports life. It is a tap into the subterranean flow of
the Way, a nipple of the Great Mother.
Access to resources held in common; the water of life, the inner
Source. The water is there for all to draw on. Source of
life-water needed by all, welling up from the depths; the
common people, common needs and strength.

Site of creative transformation.

It reaches the inner ground, where water wells up from below
to support our common life. To realise this by unceasingly toiling
for the common good – to inspire people to find ways to share,
and support each other, carried by the Bright Omens.
Inner penetration reaches to the stream and brings it to the
surface. If you only bring up mud, your rope isn't long enough.
You haven't achieved anything yet.

The underlying structure, the network.

Communicate with others, interact.

Interpenetrating and free communication.

*Adapted freely from Stephen Karcher's Total I Ching,
(2004) Sphere Paperbacks.*

The Well Books,
365, Ditchling Road, Brighton, East Sussex, BN1 6JU, U.K.
Email: thewellbooks@gmail.com

Dear Reader,

For practical homoeopathic purposes this book presents work in progress. It is not definitive. If you have comments, corrections or criticisms, write to me. If you are a homoeopath and find good use for this remedy, send the case details and your insights too; also suggestions for additions to rubrics or Materia Medica. These can all contribute to a future edition.

Thank you,

Stuart Deeks

PLASTIC WRAPPED

The Homoeopathic Proving of Cling Film

This is to give you information about
a new medicine in the homoeopathic Materia Medica.
The proving took place at the beginning of 2004.
The information has been well tested during a five year
probation period. We are now in a position to confirm
its domain and indicate its potential.

Stuart Deeks
Proving co-ordinator and Editor

With thanks

Kathy Pitt, a principal of The South Downs School of Homoe-opathy, Chichester, England – for entrusting me to do a proving with the second year students. **Those students,** and the **non-college provers** – for stepping boldly into unpredictable territories. **Their colleagues, and the homoeopaths** who were supervisors - for their careful support and observation.

Pema Sanders, homoeopath and maker of the remedy (with **Jan Mathew**) – for her patience and steadiness in typing up the provers' reports.

Debbie Hobson - for her work typing up some of my cases.

Helios Pharmacy – for supplying the tablets.

Dieter Bauer - for his early interest and his recommendation to give the fledgling remedy a probation period – the proof of the proving!

Mike Bridger, homoeopath - for his reading of the text at an early stage, and suggestions; his observations are noted in the Materia Medica.

Lindsey Farquharson, homoeopath - for her encouragement and case examples.

Yvonne Wilson and **Mary-Jane Sharratt**, provers and both now homoeopaths – for their cases.

Caroline Jurdon - homoeopath, for her proof reading and enthusiasm.

Jason Leadbitter - for his exact and friendly instruction in the chemistry and manufacture of cling film.

Solvieig Oliver and **John Jolly** - for becoming the team for presentation and final preparation of the book.

The Patients - for agreeing to have their stories included, for the benefit of others.

Contents

INTRODUCTION

My intention for this book is that it is widely read. I have attempted to present the material in a clear and comprehensible way; firstly for homoeopaths*, so that the remedy* can be prescribed for the benefit of those who need it, and then for the interested general reader to find here an insight into what may seem to be an improbable medicine*; also to engender appreciation and understanding of the method used by homoeopaths (for some two hundred years now) to test or 'prove'* medicinal substances, in order to bring them into reliable service. For all readers the case examples are instances of use of the medicine and illustrate and confirm some of its potential.

Directions into and around the text. The order of the book, apart from these introductions, follows the sequence of events, through from the initial preparation of the medicine, then the trial or 'proving'* period, and ending with case examples. The experience of the provers forms the basis of a Materia Medica* of symptoms. These derive almost entirely from the proving text, and are mostly confirmed now from clinical experience. As time passed, we added retrospective reviews from those provers who had marked reactions, and editorial comments linking cases with the proving text etc. These are indicated in italics.

Gradually, we have become more aware of the territory of this remedy, and connections with Cinderella type stories have proved relevant. However, this chronological order of presentation may not be your best route through the text.

To dip in to the cases might be a way to start, to get straight to the point and purpose of it all. Cases 1 to 4 would provide a concise and illustrative introduction. Or the Cinderella essay might be the section to whet your appetite. I suggest you consider the whole like a mobile, with its several diverse features, all dependent on a central thread. This is reflected in that each prover's experience reveals certain facets of the whole. The same applies to the cases: each person's symptoms highlight one or more of the various aspects. The whole book can be considered as a field or open space where you spend time, having a look around; so it doesn't matter which entrance you use!

There is here a rich and lively well of information. Draw on it.

An explanation of asterisked terms used, combined with an outline of the main part of the book.

Homoeopaths are people who prescribe medicines accord-ing to the principles of homoeopathy. This word was coined by Samuel Hahnemann, early on in the nineteenth century. He was a German chemist and physician. Here are two examples of the homoeopathic principle* :

1. Something heavy, a brick maybe, falls on your foot, or you stub your toe. As first reaction you might well shout OUCH! loudly, or some other more vigorous expression, then press hard on the place of impact, for relief of the pain.

2. Eating something poisonous will bring on symptoms; if it's a lethal poison, you will die. However, the symptoms in their se-quence of stages will vary considerably depending on the nature of the poison. For example the toxicity of the common foxglove *(digitalis)* includes certain effects on heart function. The homoeo-pathic principle is seen in useful action when much smaller doses of that same dangerous poison relieve particular kinds of heart conditions. It is generally acknowledged, and not just by homoeo-paths, that poisons are an essential medical resource. Hence the symbol on the cover, known as a Caduceus. This symbolises the dual aspects of a poison: what can kill or harm as poison can relieve or 'cure' as medicine.

Proving. The word itself. Homoeopaths' use of this word reflects Hahnemann's pioneering work. In German the word 'pru-fung' is used for a trial, a test, an investigation into, or examina-tion of something. In English we have the saying 'The proof of the pudding is in the eating'. Hahnemann conducted clinical trials of the medicines of his day, and our use as homoeopaths of the word 'proving', as the name used for this method of investigating medicinal effects, came directly from the German 'prufung'.

A Prover. Someone who takes part in a proving.

What is a proving? How is a proving done?

Anyone might discover the properties of a potentially medicinal substance on their own. Accidental, as well as deliberate poisoning can be like this. The symptoms provide useful indicators of the field of action of the poison. However, deliberate provings are undertaken as a safe way to provide homoeopaths with a more thorough and detailed understanding.

With this intention tablets are prepared, usually, by a homoeopathic pharmacy, from the substance to be tested. This preparation involves sequential dilution and succussion* of the original. This has to be preceeded by trituration* if the original material is insoluble in water, as is the case with cling film. In a *trituration* an insoluble solid is broken down by pounding/pulverising it with powdered milk sugar in a mortar and pestle. The chemistry of this process is generally known and used, not only in homoeopathic pharmacies. The sequence of dilutions renders an originally poisonous substance by degrees less fiercely toxic, down to the level where it can be employed judiciously as a medicinal agent. This was done by Hahnemann to reduce the intensity of experience when taking a medicine, albeit chosen homoeopathically. Along with the dilution he established the use of succussion, which he realised as essential to retain the characteristic field of action and potency* of the medicine. Succussion involves striking the phial with the liquid inside it against a hard surface, originally a leather bound book. The medicine is made and preserved in a high alcohol medium, and this is then used to medicate blank sugar/lactose or sucrose tablets.

All *potencies* used in the proving are centesimal*. This relates to how the remedies are prepared at the pharmacy: the proportion of dilution is 1 – 99 parts at each stage. This starts with one part of the original to ninety-nine of the liquid ethanol medium. This is succussed a set number of times. One part of this mix is kept for the next stage of adding 99 parts of ethanol, and succussed again. When this is done thirty times, for example, it is known as 30 C, or 30 CH; the thirtieth centesimal potency.

One person can do a proving as a trial or test to learn about a medicine, but usually and more usefully a group will be involved. One could say that there is no such thing as perfect health, but provers are required to be clear of any obvious illness at the time of the proving. Starting on the same day at an agreed time each person takes a tablet by mouth, probably repeating the dose at intervals over a few days, stopping the dosage when they begin to experience changes. Their symptoms indicate these changes. These experiences are recorded in detail for as long as evidence of the changes continues. Some changes may be immediate, others later on.

Then, after a time, the provers' information is brought together and collated. At this stage comparisons and similarities emerge, serving to clarify the scope and territory of the medicine. As can be imagined, each prover reacts to the stimulus, in part, according to their individual sensitivities and susceptibility; for example a person, who may at other times get skin eruptions or cracking, especially in cold weather, in the proving experiences beneficial changes to his cracked finger tips. Such changes relieve an already existing condition. This indicates that the person has benefited from testing the medicine, and 'needed' it in this aspect. More commonly, experiences of change will show as new and possibly uncomfortable sensations or feelings. These stay for a while and then fade away, once the initial stimulus has 'worn off'. As indicated already, tablets are only taken until changes or symptoms are noticed, and in any case only for a few days.

The group effect. It has been frequently observed, and is the case with the proving of cling film, that others involved in the process get affected without even taking the tablets; hence the contributions to the text from supervisors.

Once most of the effects have died down, the symptoms can be sorted under headings – states of mind or spirit, emotions, as well as physical symptoms. You will see that the text of the proving in this book is laid out this way.

To match each section Rubrics* are found. These might already exist in homoeopathic repertories*, in connection with other remedies, or devised freshly to match symptoms of this proving. A *Rubric* is a means of directing someone to a particular medicine. It derives from the gained knowledge of the medicine; from poisoning, proving and confirmed clinical uses. It serves as a two way signpost – pointing to and from the medicine.

Rubrics of different medicines are brought together in repertories. A *repertory* is a 'store or collection of information, instances etc.' The word comes from the Latin reperio = I find.

This gathered and collated information tells us of states and symptoms experienced by the provers since taking the tablets. Then the medicine is ready for homoeopathic clinical use.

It goes like this: a patient comes to a homoeopath in a particular state, with symptoms. The homoeopath observes closely and goes into the detail of the symptoms. Then he or she chooses a remedy according to the homoeopathic principle. It will be one that is known from its proving to have produced/induced states and symptoms similar to those presented by the patient. (All this requires skill and enough time.) The chosen medicine is given. If the patient's state and symptoms begin to change and improve, it is considered that the medicine was a good one. (The term remedy is now justified!) The choice is confirmed and the workings of the homoeopathic principle are witnessed.

Once we had experience of this remedy in clinical use, we could begin to confirm the *Materia Medica.* In Latin this simply means 'medical material'. It represents a synthesis or distillation from the study of a particular medicine, to indicate and assist its possible uses.

It is worth adding that this whole process of proving a medicine through to Materia Medica can be repeated with another group. This has been done with long established remedies like Sulphur, one of those that Hahnemann first proved two hundred years ago. Repeated provings verify and enrich the body of information: similar threads and themes emerge, with each prover's individual nature as a colouring factor.

The terms.

Medicine, remedy and drug* are sometimes confusing, and even interchangeable.

Dictionary definitions:

Medicine – 'drug, etc. for the treatment or prevention of disease, especially taken by mouth'.

Drug – 'medicinal substance'. A word with other uses and connotations.

Remedy – 'medicine or treatment', or 'a remedy for a condition'.
The verb - 'to rectify or make good'.
(Latin remedium from medeor = heal.)

Homoeopaths tend to use 'remedy' to refer to one of the substances that they might prescribe to a patient. Other disciplines are more likely to use 'medicine' or 'drug'.

CHAPTER ONE

The story of the Proving of Plastic wrap.

When I was asked to be the co-ordinator of provings at the South Downs School of Homoeopathy, I realised that here was an opportunity to find out about plastic, in one of its many forms, so that we, as homoeopaths, could use it as a medicine. Then Pema Sanders, a colleague, drew me aside when we met at the School's annual graduation ceremony to tell me that she had an idea for a proving. (No one else was to know about it at this stage.) To our mutual surprise she had the same idea as I did . . .

In 1997, together with Jan Mathew, she had prepared cling film (from Sainsbury's) to the 30 CH potency at Helios Pharmacy, and it was waiting for a conventional proving.

As well as noting down the effects on her of making up the remedy, Pema sent it to a psychic friend for a 'reading' and organised a small 'meditation' proving amongst homoeopathy students based in Saffron Walden, Essex. *See page 175.*

The first plastics, of which bakelite was the most famous, were developed before world war one, but their rapid development came in the 1930's and 1940's with the creation of nylon, polythene, PVC and terylene.

Plastics have been used increasingly since the 1950's. Some forty years later it became evident from research into marine conditions that 1) there are particles of plastics in all sea water, and 2) that the polluting residues of petroleum derived substances (like the pesticide DDT) have a hormonal (and alarming) effect on marine life. This effect was at first described as disrupting or mimicking oestrogen; now the understanding is that the chemicals do not have a hormonal function themselves but disrupt the enzymes that control oestrogen.

We chose cling film as an example of a plastic for a proving. Pema Sanders and I swapped thoughts on the likely medicinal potential of this substance.

Firstly we thought that there would be an effect on sex hormones. We shared the common suspicion that cling film, and other plastics, infiltrate the food chain through direct proximity

1

to food and drink. By analogy with the observed impact on marine life, we thought it had a hormone disrupting effect.

Because of the falling levels of sperm counts in 'Western' countries, and the possible part played in this by substances getting into the food chain, we surmised that the hormonal aspects of the remedy might relate to issues of successful conception, as well as to the 'balance' of male and female energies within an individual; also that the proving might produce (or resolve) skin symptoms, being derived from petroleum. (The homoeopathic remedy *Petroleum* finds a use in certain kinds of skin conditions.)

(Added in June 2009.) These were our thoughts before the proving. They reflect an imprecise view, as if all plastics and other substances derived from oil were having the same effect. For example Phthalates are implicated in the hormonal disruption of marine life, but are not a constituent of plastic wrap. Now, thanks to information from a chemist in the plastics industry, we have a more exact understanding of the chemistry and manufacture of cling film.

We can now speculate more justifiably as to ways in which this chemistry and production process find parallels in the proving and cases. For sure we have seen striking hormonal aspects, both in provers and those who have by now benefited from the remedy; so we can consider the possibility of connections to the chemical constituents of plastic wrap. See Appendix.

The proving group were in their second year at the college and all female, so we invited four men to take part – two of these did sperm analyses before and after. (The results turned out to be inconclusive. A larger trial is perhaps called for here?)

We had eleven provers in all. The remedies were prepared at Helios Pharmacy, Kent, England, and coded; this means that neither provers nor anyone else involved knew which potency was being taken by which prover, or who was the one person taking placebo (un-medicated lactose tablets). Otherwise the active, medicated tablets were in the 12 CH, 30 CH and 200 CH potencies. The proving began on January 22nd, 2004. The provers were to take a maximum of six tablets over two days, and to stop when symptoms began to show up, following Jeremy Sherr's proving guidelines *(see Bibliography)*.

Each prover had a 'supervisor', another student from the same college year group. The men were supervised by Pema Sanders, myself and Yvonne Morris, homoeopath. The supervisor's role was to speak with their prover, every day to begin with, and for both to keep a record. Apart from Pema Sanders and myself none of the provers or supervisors knew what the remedy was made from. The provers were Morag Bouterse, Sarah Knight, Jackie Ryan, Nicola Schilling, Mary-Jane Sharratt, Christina Weston, Yvonne Wilson, Jon Caplin, Chris Garland, Graham Love and Stephen Phillips. The college 'supervisors' and other members of the college year group were Chris Braithwaite, Jo Brookbank, Lisa Corrigan, Jane Glover, Rebecca Johnson, Lotte Katz, Tara Lavelle, Melody Pettigrew, Tony Smith and Paul Wales.

The student group met at college sixteen days into the proving, and again four weeks after that. This first group meeting and exchange of experience seemed to 're-energise' the proving. Some provers, when hearing their colleagues' accounts, realised that some of their own experiences, which they had dismissed as insignificant or coincidental, were in fact part of the proving. We also noticed that several several supervisors had been affected. *See page 78*. This phenomena has been noted in other provings. At the second college weekend the nature of the remedy was disclosed – this was now six weeks into the proving.

I hope you find value and meaning in these writings. They are deliberately extensive and inclusive. The cases, from October 2004 onwards, include much of the individual patients' own words. Cases continue to come in as I write this (May 2009). In what I have included and written I do not intend to define or limit the territory of this medicine; rather to provoke and catalyse your thoughts and responses to the matter in hand. The remedy is after all still in its infancy. Many proving symptoms have been replicated in the clinical situation: patients sometimes using the same turn of phrase as did the provers. That helps to confirm and guide the use of the remedy. These confirmed symptoms are indicated in the Materia Medica *(Chapter Six)*.

The exploration of the Cinderella/Catskin type of tales may be of interest to you. I found it a rich and fascinating study, uncovering remarkable parallels to themes that arose from both the proving and the cases.

The Provers

Prover no. 1	(F)	36 years old.	30 CH.
Prover no. 2	(F)	33	200 CH
Prover no. 3	(F)	22	12 CH
Prover no. 4	(F)	36	12 CH
Prover no. 5	(F)	41	Placebo *See page 81*
Prover no. 6	(F)	33	30 CH
Prover no. 7	(F)	25	200 CH
Prover no. 8	(M)	55	30 CH *See page 65*
Prover no. 9	(M)	62	200 CH
Prover no. 10	(M)	54	30 CH
Prover no. 11	(M)	49	12 CH

A prover's number is given at the head of each section of text.

The Rubrics

The rubrics and page numbers that follow each section of the text refer to Robin Murphy's Homeopathic Medical Repertory, Second Edition, 2003.The rubrics were worked out by Pema Sanders and myself. We include several new rubrics, indicated in *italics.* Apart from the rubrics relating to bulimia and anorexia (page 52) all the rubrics are derived from the proving information.

CHAPTER TWO

The text of the proving

MIND: states of mind and emotional responses

Under each section heading you will find those provers' diary notes that are relevant to that theme (or symptom area). Each prover is identified by a number. You will notice some similarities of response within the group as you read through a section, also themes overlapping between sections. Another 'route' through the proving text would be to follow one prover's record by number, as it shows up in the various sections. This will enable you to form an image of that person's experience as a whole. Prover number eight's text is an example of this (page 65).

You will not find provers nos. 5 and 8 in this part of the text; this is explained on pages 81 and 65. There are only a few entries for prover no. 11. It is worth noting that prover no. 3 was taking a contraceptive pill at the time; it is possible (likely?) that her experience was affected by this.

In the proving text and cases you will come across references to other medicines prescribed by homoeopaths. For more information about the nature and scope of these remedies I recommend that you ask an amenable homoeopath, or consult a general homoeopathic Materia Medica.

The rubrics for each section are presented, as is customary, with a key word first, then the rest of it as if back to front! Examples:

Fear, falling of, walking when = fear of falling when walking.
Body, general, unattractive feels = Feels generally unattractive.
Water, drinking, as if one glass of seemed many = when she had drunk just one glass of water, she felt like she had drunk lots more than that!

Remember that they are compact, pithy, verbal signposts to help homoeopaths find a particular remedy; it's a Nineteenth Century equivalent to an internet word search engine.

Vivacity, loquacity and euphoria, and the need to be the centre of attention.

1) General sense of self-centredness and wanting to be the centre of attention. (This wore off later on) Feeling of being more interesting than others, and easily bored by other people's stuff (Day 16).

3) I was enjoying work today, in a light-hearted and laid-back mood, and laughed easily. Noticeably lively after lunch, alert and giggly with work colleagues (Day 1).
I woke from talking out loud in my sleep, and I remember the word that woke me – it was "optimistic". Partner heard me laugh out loud in my sleep. My dream world last night was obviously very light-hearted (Day 5).
Lightness and spontaneity has passed now (Day 20).

4) Very happy and chatty today, on a high. Not much of a breath between words. Articulating with hands quite a bit whilst talking (Day 12).

Very chatty and friendly to everyone *(she is an airline hostess)* - good mood. I feel very energetic, lively and positive. Talked all day to colleagues. It was commented on: "Can you stop talking for a minute!?" Friends said to me that I was very chirpy and talkative, and seemed very confident (Day 13).

Still talking. Feel clear-headed, feel optimistic and excited about life in general. Relaxed and happy at home (Day 14).

Felt energetic all day and absolutely could not stop talking. Very jovial and witty, but had enormous urge to talk ALL the time. Am chatty normally, but this was constant. Extremely friendly and caring to passengers on board. This was more than usual and it didn't wear off. Also my relationship with my husband is really good – I couldn't wait to get home to see him. It's fantastic (Day 15).

Supervisor's note: She said she felt 'fantastic' (in a very loud, excited voice) – a bit like the euphoria you see on Christmas day when the child gets the toy it always wanted. She butts in on our conversation, changing the subject really quickly, and I can't keep up. She sounds as high as a kite. The kind of talking I can imagine as when someone is on speed. She is so happy, it's fantastic. (Compare with Case 12 pages 141 and 143. Ed.)

Prover again. Not so manic today. I still feel good, though not on a high. I feel OK with household duties, and am still looking forward to my husband coming home. I feel closer to my husband, and he seems really happy today (Day 16).

Supervisor's note : She had the chatters still, and was very happy and giggly. It was infectious. She is full of ideas on how to study and do things, and is very enthusiastic about them. She seemed to write as fast as she talked. Last month, after the college weekend, she was talking of giving up the course. This weekend she is buying up the pharmacy and forming ideas left right and centre. Our tutor even said there was a lot of energy in the room. It was strange, but all four of us students had the giggles 'big time', reducing us to tears often. It makes me smile just thinking of it. FANTASTIC (Day 18).

(Next day.) *I got a text message from my prover at 7.40 a.m. It reads: "HYPER, HYPER. Waiting outside for Tesco's to open. I think I'll clean the car!" She had to wait fifteen minutes in the car for Tesco's to open, and she couldn't wait, so went to the gym for a coffee. (Provers had been asked either to change their habitual coffee/tea/alcohol consumption well before the proving or to carry on as usual in this respect through the proving.) She* had been up since 6.30 a.m., bright as a button. Did loads before school. Was multi-tasking, cooking three meals at once, and going on the computer – all at the same time.

Prover again. I didn't eat breakfast or lunch, as I was just too hyper. I feel as if I'm on speed. I love the energy and life the proving has brought to me. I feel much more affectionate towards my husband, all my jobs are being done on time, i.e. bills are dealt with immediately. I feel totally hyped from the weekend. After college on Sunday I went home, I typed up all the notes and emailed them, then did loads of other college stuff.

Supervisor's comment: This is the most hyper day she has had since the start of the proving. The conversation started with her not speaking too fast, but it soon sped up till I just couldn't speak. When I did get to talk I was being interrupted because she just had to tell me what else she was talking and thinking about.

Prover again. I feel I am buzzing, and the mood seems to be infectious. My son seems hyper today too. Made lots of decisions today, which is so unlike me. I'm not thinking about what will happen when I come down; I know I've enjoyed it, and I hope I come down slowly (Day 19).

I feel back to normal. Hyper-ness has now gone, I came down slowly, and I feel more indecisive again. I still feel as though I'm being efficient.

Supervisor: She still sounds very positive and enthusiastic, just the hyper-ness has gone (Day 25).

My constant need to move around with lots of energy has subsided, but I still feel focussed, and am positive about life in general. Getting on well with husband, and home life feels very positive (Day 26).

Co-ordinator's comment: When relating my own recent experiences and dreams at the first general meeting of the group since the proving had begun, I also was very excitable, and keen (over keen?) to talk about my experience. SD.

6) *Three hours after first tablet* - Tingling sensation all over, as if excited about something. Quite a sensual feeling. Goose

bumps, butterflies in stomach, like anticipation, but for no particular reason (Day 1).
'Butterflies in stomach' sensation again, as yesterday (Day 2).

10) Have felt relaxed and generally it's been a relaxing day. Quite euphoric. I have felt excited and engaged still with the positive experience from last night, when I was leading a meditation group for the first time (Day 1).
General positivity (unusual for me) – but I had started a Buddhist teaching class at the same time as starting the proving. I had been asked to do it – for me it was a big accolade (Day 4).
Today I've had an enjoyable day, but not euphoric as on the first day (Day 5).
Still less euphoric – I feel OK and positive, but things have settled down. I think it's having an effect on my sexual energy. I feel less caught up in my sexual energy, and less likely to have a sexual fantasy. I feel sexually calmer (Day 6).
I did the meditation teaching again, but I felt nothing like as euphoric as last time – so maybe some of it was the remedy. I feel a bit deflated. Today I had a realisation of what a big thing I've taken on (the class) – I've felt overwhelmed by the realisation of the responsibility (Day 7).
Two days later - Mood change: there has been a strong change from the positivity in the last two days. I feel less sexually calm, and seeking sexual fantasy as a comfort, and less happy in myself. I've lost confidence in my meditation practice. Other areas of my life which are difficult for me are more starkly present. I feel more self-doubting.
I have strong emotional responses at the moment – perhaps I'm more open, and I'm experiencing all of this more than I would before the proving. It feels like an intensifying of yesterday's mood, and this morning I've felt quite tearful. The mood is unhappiness related to aspects of my life which present difficulty, but for which no immediate solution presents itself. Rather, I need to work within the situation, but in doing so I can become unclear as to whether I'm making appropriate decisions – that is, keeping a balance between prevarication and overreaction (Day 9).
Mood has lifted, feeling lighter and more positive (Day 10).
I think the emotional stuff at the end of last week was a bit of a climax, and now it's just in the background (Day 13).

A profuse cold started today, the first for about three years. It came on suddenly, after an intense discussion with the lodger, with whom I had had unresolved difficulties (Day 21).

Rubrics

(Page numbers as in Homeopathic Medical Repertory – Murphy)

Chapter MIND
Talking, pleasure in his own 1410
Talking, excessive 1409
Talking, excited 1410
Talking, excessive, changing quickly from one subject to another 1409
Gesticulates, while talking 1340
Speech, hasty 1400
Optimistic 1380
Excitable 1321
Vivacious 1417
Exhilaration 1324

New rubric
Mind, talking, interrupts others 1410

Enhanced perceptions

1) Maybe getting more self-aware. I'm conscious that I'm a terrible gossip at work and getting somewhat indiscreet. I feel a bit guilty about this. I'm not sure that indiscretion is a new thing, or just something I'm more aware of (Day 8).

2) *Pre-proving* - I received the remedy in the post, and for safekeeping placed it in my remedy drawer in my therapy work-room. *(She is a reflexologist.)* Since then have experienced a feeling of heightened awareness in several situations. I have become aware of, and experience, a noticeable flow of energy whilst practising healing therapies in this room.
    Then, a few days into the proving - In comparison to prior to the proving I now feel that I've lost that heightened aware-

ness and ability to channel healing energy. I can compare myself to the difference between wood and metal. Wood is dense with no conductivity, and it acts as a barrier, but metal has conductivity and allow the energy to flow. It feels as if I'm not 'plugged in'. It feels like my skin is opaque, and light cannot shine through. Looking back I feel as if I've lost a couple of days, and realise that during this time I lost all concept of time (Day 4).

4) My son's voice seems so loud, louder than normal. I visited a friend who also sounded louder than normal. I felt as if I wanted to tell her to keep her voice down – it was penetrating my ears (Day 1).

6) Sensitive to noise and odours – man in petrol station in front of me just stank. When I came through the front door, the house smelled and the dog smelled (Day 1).

9) My senses of smell and vision are more acute (Day 9).
Since the proving began I seem to be more psychic. I 'see' things more (Day 15).

10) Today I really noticed how my work affects my back (Day 1).
(He is a bodywork practitioner.)
Again I'm really noticing how my back tightens up when giving treatments (Day 4).

Rubrics

Chapter MIND
Time, perception, loss of 1414
Sensitive, noise to 1394
Sensitive, odours to 1395
Chapter HEARING
Acute, hearing, to voices and talking 995
Chapter VISION
Acute, sensitive 1891

New rubric
Chapter GENERALS
Awareness, general, heightened 751

Speaking out, sense of connectedness or separation, in everyday encounters. Embarrassment.

1) I seem to be more 'open' with people. I have an innate, well hidden shyness, that makes me feel awkward speaking to people I don't know (shop assistants, in pubs, in the supermarket queue etc.) and I think I put out an air of standoffishness. This seems to have dispersed and people seem to be speaking to me more (Day 4).
(This prover benefited some months later on from the remedy Platina.)
By now I really don't want to speak to anyone. If I didn't have to work, I'd be cocooned at home in safety. It's OK doing usual stuff, because I know that and it's familiar, but I don't want to get out and meet new people particularly. I should have phoned my supervisor today but I don't want to. I'm bored of talking about myself and my symptoms (Day 12).
See also her headache details on Days 11 and 12. Page 34.

2) Today I was slow in talking and thinking. However, I had a very lucid conversation at the school gate about a friend's daughter, and was more outspoken than I would usually be (Day 2).
Feelings of insecurity like an outcast or an alien. When at the supermarket till, I realise I'd forgotten an item and go to get it; then I have an extreme feeling as though everyone is looking at me (Day 3).
Feelings of being lonely and separate from everybody else. A sense of unhappiness and comparing myself to other people. "I'm not a bad person, why am I not happy?" (Day 5).
See Prover number two's extra proving notes, page 75.

3) Felt cheerful at work, but strangely, alongside this was a sense of uneasiness when alone talking with another person. Then I was not as confident as when I am in a group. Felt unsociable and quite uneasy about being approached for a conversation when working alone in one of the offices. Uncomfortable and awkward, and unable to hide this. I flushed with embarrassment and realisation that I was not showing the same friendly part of myself that I had earlier. This must be an anxiety/insecurity deep within myself – yet it annoyed me that I was unable to avoid feeling this way. I've noticed that the

simplest exchanges of communication are a hurdle to get through calmly at times. Yet at other times I'm so sociable, and open enough to feel really good about myself, and feel good generally (Day 12).

With my partner I felt as though we were closely bonding for the first time in ages, and a closeness was rekindled. I felt very at ease (Day 22).

Understanding from people and being able to communicate on the same wavelength is better at work and at college, but not with my boyfriend (Day 27).

4) More open to asking questions at college – normally feel embarrassed that the question may sound silly. Today felt it didn't matter (Day 17).

Felt much more energetic today, more confident in class, asking questions and participating more than normal (Day 18).

6) I've noticed an emotional change today – over the last few weeks I have been feeling quite isolated and have had difficulty making contact with people (face to face, or by telephone). This feeling is gone today. I feel more open towards people, and people seem to be more welcoming, not so hostile – which I had felt them to be before the proving.

Went out with partner and friends for an evening meal. Under the influence of a little alcohol (two glasses of wine with food), I had a big, loud argument with my partner. Stood up, shouted at him, threatened to leave him. This is not the kind of thing I have ever done before. I felt terribly upset, but in hindsight I wonder whether my reaction was as justified as I thought at the time. It was quite out of character. It is not how I normally act, at home or in public; I tend to go quiet instead (Day 3).

Thoughts about my general state of mind – I'm a day or two away from getting my period, usually this means quite an emotional state – very irritable, very tired, no energy, no motivation etc. However, this time I feel quite balanced. I have noticed very short-lived mood swings: feeling fed-up one minute, feeling very tired, want to sit down, exhausted ... five minutes later I'm full of enthusiasm and energy. Generally I'm feeling quite good, fairly balanced, more open towards people, more easily ready to talk to people I don't know. More able to make an effort rather than feeling trapped inside myself, which I usually feel quite strongly when pre-menstrual (Day 16).

Rubrics

Chapter MIND
Bashful 1282
Reserved 1386
Timid 1415
Anxiety in company 1272
Anxiety from conversation 1272
Embarrassment, feelings of 1320

New rubric
Estranged, feels, while going about her daily business 1284

Chapter DELUSIONS
Separated from the world 375
Looking at her, everyone is 371
Alone, world, that she is alone in the 360

Cleaning up, tidiness, washing.

1) I had a dream about my neighbour – she came to say the remedy I gave her didn't work. I had to retake the case, and was fairly obsessed with the fact that she is tidy. In my dream that was important.

I seem to be neat the past two days, keeping things tidy in the house, but I do have phases like that – if it persists, it is definitely the remedy. 8 p.m., still tidying up, although its evening (Day 2).

I'm still tidying up at every opportunity – I was ironing at 9 p.m. – not usual (Day 3).

Was desperate to do some washing – although there was none in the basket! I cleaned the kitchen windows this morning – very unusual. Also I turned down my socks neatly, which is unusual too (Day 4).

I asked my partner if I'm still tidy and he said "Yes". It's becoming such a part of me, I no longer notice. Usually it's a mad rush getting the house tidy on Thursday mornings for the cleaner - but today it was already tidy. At work I've cleared up all loose ends and finished up outstanding jobs, but oddly, I don't feel as though I've worked particularly hard this week. I've a project to work on, so we'll get on with that today. My tidiness at home has extended to tidying up loose ends at work too, I think (Day 8). House seems dusty, and I plan to give it a good clean, even the windows. Evidently, tidiness continues. *Later in the day* - I can't believe the last three hours have gone so fast. I've been having a cleaning frenzy – hoovering the stairs, changing the sheets, polishing the kitchen floor (I can't remember when I last did that), cleaning windows, and hand-washing stuff. Its helped my period pain! I'm not sure why I can't stop cleaning and tidying, we're not having visitors, so it's not out of necessity. I just want the space around me to be clean. I can't bear any dirt or untidiness at the moment (Day 10).

Definitely less tidy today, and have eaten more, and less 'good' food (Day 11).

In retrospect (after the proving) - About three and a half weeks into the proving I felt clearer and cleaner. I felt more attractive, and was noticing men's attractiveness.

4) Needed to tidy house before college (Day 17).

Rubrics

Chapter   MIND
Tidy   1414
Fastidious   1326
Fastidious, for cleanliness   1326

New rubric
Housekeeping, attentive to   1345

Precise detail

1) I got into a debate about apostrophes, which is the one grammatical thing I'm not good at. I felt I was on weak ground, and didn't have the confidence to argue a convincing case (Day 4).

3) My partner said I've gone into a lot more detail about things generally since the proving began. He felt I'd been more descrip-

tive than necessary to explain myself (Day 3).
I agree with my partner that I am 'going into one' about detail even more often than usual (Day 5).

4) As I look around I feel as if I'm looking at everything in detail (Day 15).

Rubrics

Chapter MIND
Fastidious, details for   1326

Organisation and overwhelm. Motivation and procrastination.

1) It will be interesting to see if I get on with 'put off' jobs at work tomorrow and feel more motivated (Day 4).
I've got lots of bits done at work, but not yet knuckled down to the project I'm supposed to be doing. I was quite quiet today, not sure if this is the remedy, or just me. I don't usually feel like this. I need to phone a couple of tradesmen, but keep putting it off – not sure why. I just don't feel up to it somehow. A few years ago I'd put off phoning friends until I felt in the right mood, and I suppose this is similar. Also I notice I've been walking more slowly today, not in a rush, and it seems to suit my slightly withdrawn mood (Day 20).

2) Initially I felt motivated, going out on several trips, completing jobs I'd been meaning to do for ages; it was like when I was pregnant: I felt happy, motivated and energetic. However, by now I feel tired, lethargic, mentally dull and confused. I had a couple of minor near-miss errors while driving. I felt slow, dreamlike – it was really hard to get my mind into gear. I've felt mentally dull, almost as if drunk, and time seemed distorted. As the afternoon went on I felt it hard to manage everyday tasks, and felt overwhelmed by work. I had to work really hard to complete a small piece of written work (this is unusual), although there were no mistakes in it when it was checked by my colleague. My brain felt swollen/waterlogged. I was confused and was making mistakes in talking and completing tasks, e.g. made a cheese sauce but forgot

to cook the pasta (Day 1).
Realised I have not completed many tasks I had planned to do —
tidying, clearing etc (Day 2).

3) *Prover's overview* – Since the proving began I have had a sense
of pressing and reminding of things I want to do. Before, I would
wait. Now I would do it now. All those things I was going to do
if I wasn't going to be criticised, judged or doubted. Life is too
short — what is the most pressing thing you would do if this was
your last day? Before I would make plans, wanting something to
look forward to, rather than be just 'in the now' (Day 28).

4) I feel positive and motivated, clear head, feeling focussed (Day 1).
I really enjoyed cooking dinner, I wouldn't normally. I seem more
focussed, and not indecisive. Instead of sitting about and moaning about things I'm actually getting on with it. Achieved quite a
bit. I've got a positive attitude. I'm getting more done (Day 4).
I feel really positive about everything (Day 8).
All my jobs have been done on time — bills have been dealt with
immediately. Absolutely hyper today — jumped out of bed at
6 a.m. full of energy. Felt as though I'd taken amphetamines.
Tidied house, and was waiting outside Tesco's to do shopping at
7.45 a.m. — it didn't even open till 8 a.m. Went to two supermarkets, came home, made three different soups and two other
meals, and cleaned the house. Forgot to eat breakfast and lunch,
as I could not stop moving. Accomplished everything I had been
meaning to do today, very focussed, did not slow down until going
to bed at midnight. Slept well. I made a lot of decisions today,
which is very unlike me. I'm not thinking about what will happen
when I 'come down'. I know I've enjoyed it, I hope I come down
slowly (Day 19).
Did a lot of work on the house today, painting outside with husband — getting on well, feeling very together. Calm and relaxed,
not energetic any more. I enjoyed feeling so lively, I miss it. I
accomplished many unfinished jobs during the proving. I feel back
to normal now, though still feel it has left me very positive and
organised. I feel optimistic about the course, and can see homoeopathy as part of my future. I had many doubts before, that
I could cope with the course, and always felt as if I could give it
up. I've not had this feeling again since the proving (Day 25).

10) Today I made one very quick decision, which is unusual for me. I just saw this form that I had to fill in, filled it in, and made out a cheque, and that was it! (Day 1).

11) Felt 'on form' today, achieved a lot at work without feeling stressed (Day 1).
Felt good again today, mentally (Day 2).
Felt good all day again, a general feeling of changing up into fifth gear. Its like going into overdrive. I'm going as fast as before, although it doesn't feel I have to work as hard to maintain the speed (Day 3).
A bit stressed today, not quite as relaxed as before (Day 7).
Feeling stressed again (Day 8).
Head clear again (Day 12).
Last night I had a 'down' mood for about an hour – no reason for it, not too stressed at work etc. – but suddenly felt 'fed-up' with everything – where I'm going in my life etc. Glum moodiness, 'poor me', tearful over nothing in particular. My gums were bleeding, my piles were bleeding, and I felt moody, almost like a woman with PMT. It went as suddenly as it came! Looking back over the last three weeks – I have been functioning better with my academic work, in general (Day 22).

Rubrics

Chapter MIND
Worries, full of 1421
Business, incapacity for 1284
Undertakes many things, perseveres in nothing 1416
Workaholic 1420
Procrastinates 1381
Gloomy 1341

New rubric
Gloomy, motivation without 1342

Calmness and focus

1) At work, one of my clients by-passed me and went straight to one of the directors. Usually this would piss me off, but it didn't today. I just phoned him and had a quick discussion about what he wanted. I was much more relaxed about stuff than I used to be (Day 5).

3) On the journey home by car I was content to leave the car radio off, and just to reflect on my day. This is not usual for me (Day 1).
Silence is now too much again, so I have to have music on (Day 20).
This evening I just wanted to watch the film we chose in silence, which is unlike me, as I have often been told off for talking my way through films, much to everyone's annoyance (Day 25).

4) I feel really chilled out, like really relaxed. Lost my purse at work today, but was really calm about it, wasn't bothered. A lack of usual reactions to things. It feels like being stoned. I feel as if I have more patience than normal with my son. I spoke very calmly to him in the supermarket as he was really being boister-ous and loud. I kept very together even though his voice was tiring me out. I cooked dinner and answered his millions of ques-tions very responsibly – which is often not so easy when tired at the end of the day. I did start to raise my voice and lose control slightly when preparing him for bed (Day 1).
Still feel more patient than usual with my son (Day 4).
Don't feel as relaxed and calm today – feel pissed off that I am feeling like this. Feeling pissed off with the proving – knowing me I've got the placebo. My period isn't due for one week, so it isn't PMT.
Feel like doing nothing this evening, cancelled evening out with friends (Day 5).
Feel very clear headed and focussed. Calmness at home is still there. Normal situations that would wind me up just don't (Day 15).
Again very energetic, woke up refreshed at 6 a.m. – cleaned house (not normal), prepared roast dinner before 8.30 a.m., then cycled to the gym, five minutes faster than normal. Felt I had excess energy to burn, felt light and buzzing during the class,

even went to the supermarket, all before 9 a.m. Came home, did lots of other chores. Not getting wound up about domestic affairs and things that need doing – just relaxing and getting on with everything. I'm certainly more clear headed and not so fuzzy – I feel great! Working on computer at 10.15 p.m., by this time I'm normally tired and can't wait to go to sleep – not today! My main feeling normally is "I'll do it tomorrow" – now I feel I'll do everything now. Becoming more organised and feeling calmer, and not so impatient with trivia, e.g. installing programme into computer fairly calmly and not becoming irritated if I've done something wrong. Feeling as if I can sit calmly, analyse what I need to do, and then do it, without the unnecessary fuss I normally make (Day 20).

Woke up refreshed at 6 a.m. Calming down – feel very focussed, doing lots of chores, feel the urge to sort everything out – paperwork and housework – to organise everything. Not feeling so hyper. Slightly agitated with husband, because I feel I'm doing everything (Day 21).

Not much to say today, calming down, not feeling the urge to rush everything. More tired than usual (Day 22).

Felt tired today and slept all morning, as my son is staying with his grandparents. Bliss! Really relaxing – feel content (Day 23).

Still feeling friendly, chatty and calm (Day 25).

Still not irritable with household things and husband (Day 36).

6) Feel irritable and impatient with my daughter, but also calmer in reaction to situations (Day 1).

I feel more efficient, my thoughts organise easier, and I'm more focussed. I find writing essays a lot easier (Day 16).

7) Have been in a really good, cheery, light mood all day. It's been sunny with blue skies, which made me feel wonderfully relaxed. In some ways I've noticed I've been a lot more relaxed and laid-back. I had friends over for dinner and getting things ready was a bit rushed, but I felt a lot calmer when normally I'd get flustered (Day 3).

Rubrics

Chapter MIND
Tranquillity, serenity 1415
Patience 1380
Impatience 1349
Clear, mind 1287
Agitation, mental 1264

New rubric
Quiet, around her, cannot stand 1382

**Sadness, self-doubt, and feeling withdrawn.
Sensitive to the opinion of others.**

1) I've not felt this sad for years. I have no appetite, but managed to force some lunch down. It's a general flatness and sad feeling. I was on a train, and a mother was threatening to hit her little boy – I couldn't see that he was doing anything wrong – just being a lively five year old. Another person had a run-in with a ticket inspector. Right now I don't want to be surrounded by all of this, and I wish they'd all go away (Day 16).
I feel a bit 'hunched-up' and closed in on myself today. A friend said I looked tired. I need to phone a couple of tradesman, but keep putting it off, not sure why, just don't feel up to it somehow. I've also noticed that I've been walking more slowly today, not in a rush, and it seems to suit my slightly withdrawn mood (Day 20).

2) I felt very sad, alone and insecure (Day 2).
Feel shaky, sick, insecure, paranoid, withdrawn, sad and lonely. I cannot be bothered to talk and make conversation (Day 3).
The next day - In the afternoon I went to a children's party. I felt sick on the way. The paranoid, withdrawn, insecure feeling came back. I feel very sensitive, I feel like I'm doing things wrong. The sun is shining, but I feel very sad and alone. I feel particularly sensitive to the opinions of others. I feel that if I was a better person, everything would be better. I had a panic attack at the party – very mild, but it felt like I couldn't breathe. I managed to keep it to myself. When I came home I felt better, but there was still a sick feeling there, and I didn't have any dinner. I still have a shaky feel-

ing, and I am still making some mistakes. I wish this feeling would go . . . (Day 4).

The withdrawn feeling is less today, but I still feel insecure, worried and anxious (Day 5).

Worried, insecure feeling is back again. A lot of self-doubt, and I've felt sad. I have the sense of others' happiness again, and the lack of it in myself. This feeling was still there at 6 p.m., but it eased off during the evening (Day 6). *Supervisor's observation - She realised that she had been experiencing contradictory feelings about situations: caring, but not caring; worried, but not worried. She feels as if an insecure side of her character has been exposed.*

4) I don't feel at all sociable today – I can't be bothered with talking. Everything is a real effort (Day 11).

Usually I have feelings of doubt about college work - negative thoughts like "I'm not good enough" or "I can't do it". Since the proving began I don't have these thoughts. I feel confident and positive (Day 17).

10) Mood change: there has been a strong change from the positivity in the last two days. I feel less sexually calm, and seeking sexual fantasy as a comfort, and less happy in myself. I've lost confidence in my meditation practice. Other areas of my life which are difficult for me are more starkly present. I feel more self-doubting (Day 9).

Rubrics

Chapter MIND
Depression, sadness 1308
Depression, sadness, company, aversion to, desire for solitude
1308
Depression, sadness, happy on seeing others 1309
Depression, sadness, quiet 1311
Depression, sadness, talk, indisposed to 1311
Confidence, lacking, no self-esteem 1290
Loneliness 1367
Isolation, feelings 1360
Panic, attacks of anxiety 1380
Chapter DELUSIONS
Right, does nothing 375

Clumsiness and cautiousness

1) I felt clumsy, and banged my head. Later I went for a walk and fell over in the mud (Day 4).

2) I felt clumsy, nearly dropped a cup of hot tea. I managed to catch it, but it splashed everywhere (Day 1).

6) Quite nervous and apprehensive about the snowfall, and indecisive about what action to take re the school run. I decided to go a little later, when maybe the roads will have cleared. Very agonised by this inconvenience, which is unusual – normally I would not take it so seriously. Later when walking in town, I avoid crossing the road, because there is snow and ice on the other side. Usually this would not bother me to this extent – I would wobble across the ice without a second thought. I'm worried about falling, and don't normally feel like that. I seem to be very cautious (Day 8).

Rubrics

Chapter MIND
Awkward, mentally, drops things 1281
Fear, falling of, walking when 1330
Cautious 1284
Cautious, anxiously 1284

Mental confusion

1) *An hour after the first tablet* - When driving to work I feel a bit vague, and keep gazing into the middle distance with a blank mind. I forgot to indicate when turning right – it is an effort to make myself do this (Day 1).

2) By early evening I had the feeling as if I was drunk on water – my brain felt swollen/waterlogged. I was confused and was making mistakes in talking and in completing tasks, for example I made a cheese sauce, and forgot to cook the pasta. My memory was also affected – I was losing the thread of what I was talk-

ing about, stopping midway through what I was saying, pausing, and then repeating the last few words I had just said but still not finishing the sentence. I was aware I was doing this, but didn't seem stressed by it. I didn't like feeling dazed like this (Day 1).

As yesterday, continue to feel dazed – I felt mentally numb. I had to concentrate hard when driving my son to school. I was slow in talking and thinking. Realised I had double-booked things in my diary yesterday. My memory is poor, my speech is slow and confused, and I feel like I'm struggling to do even one thing at a time – when I can usually manage five. Time seems distorted, and I find myself staring into space (Day 2).

The following morning I enjoyed being out in the sunshine – I feel better in the fresh air. My speech and thought are more connected and lucid when in the fresh air.

Later on I noticed that I was unable to do more than one thing at a time, and by 10.30 a.m. I felt dazed again. I feel slow, quiet and tired. I'm still making mistakes, my memory is bad, I can't judge time at all and keep having to look at the clock. Later on I felt a bit better, but was still making mistakes – I wore my watch in the shower, and when cooking threw the mushrooms away and kept the stalks. The 'waterlogged brain' feeling is still there, and slight headache. It's as if my brain is too big for my skull – a sense of fullness in my head (Day 3).

The next day - This morning I have the 'waterlogged brain' feeling again, although I have not drunk much water. I feel really tired and dazed. Still have the shaky feeling, and still making some mistakes (Day 4).

Felt sick, shaky, nervous feeling, and overwhelmed by the day ahead. When I took my son to school I still felt jumpy and on edge. My memory is still really bad – I can't remember what arrangements I've made over the last few days. I realised I haven't kept up with people, haven't phoned people back, or replied to emails over the last few days (Day 5).

Memory still bad, easily overloaded mentally – I've felt like this all day (Day 6).

Appetite fine, no feeling of nausea, and am feeling more positive. Feelings of sadness, self-doubt and anxiety have all gone, but my memory is still bad. I still find it hard to concentrate on several tasks. I'm easily overwhelmed mentally and find it really hard to spell (Day 7).

Still feeling mentally overwhelmed by small things. My memory is still really bad. At lunchtime I get the 'waterlogged' feeling in my head again, as if drunk on water, although I had not drunk much. It's hard to concentrate, and I'm slow to react.
My co-ordination is slow (Day 8).
I have an ongoing problem with awareness of time – it's as if time passes too quickly. I have to keep checking my watch for the time – in particular this applies to therapy sessions – because I'm unable to judge the passing of time (Day 10).
On occasions I still have to look at my watch in therapy sessions, when in the past I had an intuitive sense of the passage of time (Day 19).

3) *Prover's review* - I believe that my general state of confusion is connected with the fact that I'm confusing my body, and therefore myself, by being on the Pill. During the proving I felt quite disconnected from my partner at times, I had difficulties in communicating with friends at work, and found it difficult to prioritise my college homework.

6) When I discussed what my partner had said to upset me he couldn't remember saying it, and the memory is hazy for me too. I don't know what really happened – I normally remember things like this (Day 3). *See her text on page 13.*

Rubrics

Chapter MIND
Absentminded, preoccupied 1261
Concentration, general, difficult 1289
Concentration, general, difficult, can't fix attention 1289
Confusion, mental 1291
Dullness, mental 1317
Memory, general, forgetful 1370
Memory, general, weakness of 1371
Mistakes, general, time in 1375
Speech, finish sentence, cannot 1400
Speech, general, slow 1401
Time, perception, loss of 1414
Time, perception, loss of, quickly passes too 1414

Concepts of time

1) *One hour after the first tablet* - Everyone seems to be driving too fast, and dangerously – this is worrying. I feel like I did when first learning to drive twenty years ago – I feel the world is going too fast. It's as if I'm gazing into 'forever' (Day 1).
Thought I would be late for work, so drove very fast- totally different from the morning of starting the proving, when I felt like a learner driver. Today I caught myself driving too fast (Day 3).

2) Aware now of regularly looking at my watch to keep up with the passage of time – before I could judge half an hour accurately without having to look at my watch (Day 4).

Rubric

Chapter DELUSIONS
Time, space, and/or lost and confused 378

Spaced out and ungrounded

1) 10 a.m. Feel a bit 'air-headey', not quite grounded, a bit vague. *Later* - Have eaten lunch and feel better, more grounded (Day 1).

4) I feel really chilled-out, like really relaxed. A lack of my usual reactions to things. It feels like being stoned (Day 1).

Rubric

Chapter MIND
Spaced-out feeling 1399

Effects of alcohol, sensations as if drunk.

1) *Two hours after the first tablet* - My eyes feel a bit fuzzy, and I don't seem to have total control of my movements, a bit like being slightly drunk or tipsy (Day 1).
No desire for alcohol this evening - unusual for a Friday night! (Day 2).
Energy levels feel good – better than usual. Might be helped by no alcohol, but I didn't even want to drink last night – I felt I would be drunk after just one glass (Day 3).
Had a curious feeling of lightness in bed last night, my headache was gone, and I realised that alcohol really is my 'poison'. I didn't drink last night and I think that even just one drink in general makes me feel worse. It's even worse for me than cigarettes. Maybe I'm more self-aware at the moment (Day 10).
Review (Day 16). General aversion to alcohol for the past two weeks, no desire to drink.
Four weeks later – Still no desire to drink.

2) 2 p.m. I felt slow, and dreamlike – it was really hard to get my mind in gear and I felt mentally dull, almost drunk. Time seems distorted. By late afternoon/early evening I felt nauseous and had a slight frontal headache – the whole feeling was as if I was drunk on water (Day 1).
After walking the dogs I sat down for a while – felt almost anaesthetised/drunk. Felt happy, slow, spaced-out and tidy. I feel like I appeared relaxed, but felt confused. In the evening had a glass of wine, although I felt like I already had had too much. The feeling I had after drinking the wine was exactly the opposite to my normal reaction to two glasses of wine. Had been feeling very tempted to take an extra dose of the remedy all evening/late afternoon. I was using all my willpower NOT to take another tablet – the feeling was so strong. I just felt so tempted to 'top up' the feeling again. I resisted the temptation, and had a glass of wine instead, and then felt slightly better. I had a second glass and felt sharper and more 'with it'. It was as though the effects of the remedy were reversed (Day 2).
Realised I had not been drinking as much water as usual, and in fact am quite thirstless. I had a drink of water to rectify the

situation, but this just aggravated the swimming sensations in my head. Brain feels waterlogged again, although have not drunk very much water at all. Feeling slow again, slightly dazed, unable to do more than one thing at a time. When I've only had one glass of water it feels like I've drunk loads (Day 3).

Alcoholic drinks do not seem to dehydrate me, as they would normally (Day 7).

At lunchtime I got the waterlogged feeling in my head again – drunk on water, although I have not drunk much. Even small drinks of water bring on a fuzzy head, as though I've drunk too much (Day 8).

Prover's review - Overall during the proving I found myself with a lack of thirst. Normally I can down two pints in one go, and still feel thirsty – so I would be drinking water out of habit, although I soon felt as though I had drunk too much. On one occasion I felt drunk on water, and this improved by drinking some alcohol.

3) I had a hangover when I hadn't drunk a lot. This was exaggerated compared to previous experience. I felt irritable and uncomfortable from a persistent headache (Day 26).

4) Had two sips of a gin and tonic on arriving home, felt really dizzy – as if I had drunk far more. Had to move position – I sat down on the couch, and felt weak, and then had to lie down in bed. I fell asleep (Day 10).

Alcohol seems not as appetising, so I'm drinking less (Day 22).

Rubrics

Chapter FOOD
Alcohol, general, agg. 724
Alcohol, general, aggravates, easily intoxicated 724
Alcohol, general, aversion to, alcoholic stimulants 724
Alcohol, general, desires 724
Chapter TOXICITY
Alcohol, general, agg. 1857
Alcohol, general aggravates, easily intoxicated. 1857
Alcohol, general, aversion to   1857
Alcohol, general, desires 1857

Chapter MIND
Intoxicated, sensation as if 1356
Confusion, intoxicated as if 1292

New rubric
Intoxicated, sensation as if, water from drinking 1356

Sensations and some dreams relating to water

1) In another dream the Downs *(hills in Sussex)* had lots of woodland and cattle grids, and I was riding my bike through the woods. All the fields above Brighton were flooded, and I had to swim through one field with my bike (Day 10).

2) Within five minutes of taking the first tablet I was experiencing energy waves, and a warm sensation in my lower back. It feels as if my right foot is standing in warm water. I thought something had been spilt on the floor.
Six hours later - Warm/hot feet sensations continuing – it feels like I've got my foot in hot water (Day 1).
Had several dreams, difficult to recall except for one, but they all included references to water. I dreamt of being with my mother in a building with a large swimming pool. She had heavy make-up on the left side of her face only, none on the right side. I told her that the side without make-up was better. Other dreams had dishes of water evaporating in them (Day 2).
I feel like I've drunk loads of water, but I've only had one glass (Day 3).
At lunchtime I got the waterlogged feeling in my head again – as if drunk on water, although I had not drunk much. Even small drinks of water bring on a fuzzy head, as though I'd drunk too much (Day 8).
Prover's review - Through the proving I noticed a lack of thirst. I was drinking out of habit, because normally I can down two pints in one go and still feel thirsty. Although when I did drink, I thought I'd drunk too much. On one occasion I felt drunk on water, and this improved by drinking some alcohol.

6) For three evenings now I have the sensation that my feet are ice-cold. It feels like they're in ice-cold water (Day 3).

Rubrics

Chapter DELUSIONS
Water 380

New rubric
Water, drinking, as if one glass of seemed many 365

Body image; attractiveness; relationship with others.

1) Had a dream involving a woman who worked for the Body Shop, showing me lots of photos of her in terrible sequinned clothes at various events (Day 2).
Lots of dreams – busy, loads of things going on. My brother's girlfriend refusing to get out of bed (this is quite common); people jumping off London Bridge; some good-looking man flirting with me – I can't recall any pattern (Day 3).
A dream involving a successful rock star who was flirting with me. We were attracted, but I had my partner, and he was married to someone whose name wasn't pronounced as it was spelt. I felt flattered and attractive in the dream (Day 7).
In one dream I had two dates with cute men, and got in such a muddle trying to please them, and flit between them. I just made a mess of it (Day 10).
In spite of cold and cough I feel pretty good, and also feel attractive. I've felt like this for much of the past few days – as though I have a pretty face, and am attractive (Day 27).
Prover's comment - There have been definite times since the proving began when I've felt clearer and cleaner, and more attractive. I've also noticed men's attractiveness. During sex I have felt greater intensity, more passion, and very good afterwards. My partner also seems to have been the same, and not tired the following day. But there has been no increase in the frequency of sex.

2) I feel sensitive to the opinions of others (Day 4).
I felt attractive today, which is unusual for me (Day 7).
3) I'm unhappy with how my nails look, and can't wait till they

grow back. I'm very conscious of not being attractive with nails like this (Day 10).

4) Relationship with my husband is really good. I couldn't wait to get home and see him. It's fantastic! (Day 15).
I've been looking at my husband and noticing how well he looks. A cycle seems to have been broken here. I'm so much happier, so he is happier, so there's less arguing. I feel great about this. When you're happy you don't notice the niggling things in your relationship. My husband told me I was really nice today – I wished I was like this more often. I felt loving towards him, more affectionate (Day 15).

6) Feeling a bit low – I probably spent three hours at the hairdressers, and came out looking no different, or else worse! (Day 1).

7) *Prover's review* - My breasts have grown quite a lot since the proving began. I haven't felt any more attractive, but have felt sometimes a bit 'tarty' as my breasts got bigger. I didn't write these changes down to begin with as I was already feeling some tenderness prior to the proving.

11) Since the proving began it seems that my wife has been more loving and affectionate, and noticing me more (Day 22).

Rubrics

Chapter MIND
Affectionate 1264

New Rubric
Chapter DELUSIONS
Body, general, unattractive feels 362

Weight gain or loss

1) A dream in which I was very fat (Day 2).
I felt 'fat' all morning, and trousers are too tight (Day 5).
Weighed myself today and found I've lost two pounds since start-ing the proving a week ago (Day 8).

2) Have lost three pounds in weight since the proving began (Day 6).
See also her review. Pages 76 & 77.

4) Around the time of my period I have maintained a steady weight, which is unusual for me (Day 36).

Co-ordinator (SD) I gained seven pounds in weight during the proving. (I did not take any tablets.) This established a new nor-mal weight for me, which remained so two years later.

New rubrics
Included to reflect our clinical experience of the remedy to date (Summer of 2009). For an example see Case 4.
Chapter MIND
Weight, sensitive about 1418
Weight, thinks she is too 'fat' when not overweight 1418

CHAPTER THREE

Symptoms of various parts of the body. Modalities.

Headaches

1) Headache worse as evening progressed, < alcohol, > firm pressure on temples, > bowel movement (Day 3).
9.30 a.m. Headache – dull aching. I don't often get headaches. It feels a bit like a hangover, but one and a half glasses of wine last night isn't sufficient to cause it. Headache isn't crippling, but makes me feel I want to go back to bed; I've drunk plenty of water as usual, so don't think its dehydration. 10.45 a.m. Headache is gone (Day 6).
Two days later – Have slight headache this morning, like a hangover. I did feel thirsty in the night, but somehow didn't want to wake up enough to take a drink. Headache this afternoon; in fact most of today it's been around in the background, < chocolate, I think. Thirsty today also – have drunk two litres of water and

two cups of tea just at work.

Just did a bit of Reiki to clear headache, and some eye exercises, which has helped a lot. A bit of tension in back of neck and shoulders. Headache is worse wearing glasses – I feel they are weighing down on nose and behind ears (Day 8).

The next day - Woke up this morning with cracking head, and felt so tired. Headache persisted all morning – a bit better from fresh fruit juice, < noise.

In general headache is better tilting head to right, and pressing on right temple. It is < right side and around right eye, but moves around – back of head, temple, eye, vertex. Quite piercing, but then that subsides and its just a dull ache for a few minutes until pain returns. It is as close as I've ever got to a migraine. Although the drink didn't help, I don't feel alcohol is the total cause. Also I had chocolate mousse last night, and wonder if that might be a factor. Chocolate does seem to aggravate my headaches this week. I've had more headaches this week than in the last year. I rarely get them normally. This afternoon I did thirty minutes meditation and then slept for an hour; headache had just about gone when I woke. I feel pale and a bit needy now, almost tearful, and totally worn out by the pain of the headaches, and maybe by my period too (Day 9).

Two days later - 12.00 midday. I'm developing a headache and it started behind my eyes. In the sun my eyes felt sensitive and a bit 'stiff', so it hurt when I moved them from side to side. Headache is in the top of my head and whilst not really severe, it's just there. 7.30 p.m. Headache is gone, and even chocolate hasn't affected it. I had a go at my partner earlier, and a few tears – I felt we weren't doing enough together. Maybe headaches were a symptom of bottling it up. I feel better for it, and we had a good afternoon together (Day 11).

The next day - Headache developed this afternoon, again it was right sided, behind eyes, and whole side of head. Felt as though it was full of pressure, tension; if it could explode it would feel better. It also goes down into my neck and shoulder. I ate some biscuits this afternoon and it could have been that that brought it on. It got better after I had an argument with my partner (Day 12).

Another student at college made a connection between my headaches and the time of my period, which I hadn't considered (Day 19).

3) Day one of my period – felt noticeable hot flushes all day today and a feeling of undeniable pressure all round my head – which made me feel groggy (Day 13).

Awoke feeling very groggy and with a dull headache. Overwhelming headache, distracted from it by going out for a meal (Day 23).

Hangover when I hadn't drunk a lot and this is exaggerated compared to previously. Irritable and uncomfortable from a persistent headache (Day 26).

The subtlest of headaches in the temples (Day 27).

6) *Five and a half hours after the first dose* - Headache, slight, throbbing. *An hour and a half later* - Took second dose, and headache went off for ten minutes. *Fifteen minutes after that -* Headache back.

Evening - Headache is getting worse; I don't get headaches very often (Day 1).

The next day, midmorning – Slight headache, throbbing.

Evening – Headache is still with me, and it's getting worse, really throbbing, extends into ear. 11 p.m. – Headache still very strong. I realised that the headaches tend to be worse 7 p.m. onwards (Day 2).

Two days later - Woke up with headache. When I went outside, even with a woolly hat on, it did not feel any better; this would normally help a headache. Slight headache on and off throughout the day, but not as painful as before; sometimes also pain in my neck. 10 p.m. Still with slight headache (Day 4).

No headache in the morning. Headache for one hour in the afternoon, but not as bad as before (Day 5).

No headache (Day 6).

Headache still gone (Day 8).

Rubrics

Chapter – HEADACHE
Alcohol, spiritous liquors from 907
Intoxication, after, as if 934
Menses, during 937
Noise, from 941
Pressure, external, amel. 959
Right, sided 960

Stool after, amel. 975
Sharp pain, temples, right 967
Sharp pain, temples 967
Temples, extending to neck 984
Wandering pains 993
Temples, pressure amel. 984
Pressing pain, pressure amel. 950
Temples, right side 984
Throbbing 985
Throbbing, evening 986
Evening 923

New rubrics
Pressure of glasses aggravates 959
Right sided, leaning head to right side amel. 960

Eyes

1) *Two hours after the first dose* - My eyes feel a bit fuzzy, and I don't seem to have total control of my movements. A bit like being slightly drunk or tipsy. During the morning a work colleague said my eyes look tired and glassy (Day 1).
My headache is worse on the right side, and around my right eye – but it moves around – eye, to back of head, to temple, to vertex. In general the headache is better tilting the head to the right, and pressure applied to the right temple (Day 9).
I'm developing a headache, and also reacting to sunlight. The headache started behind my eyes. In the sun my eyes felt sensitive, and a bit 'stiff', so it hurt when I moved them from side to side (Day 11).
I look tired this morning around my eyes, although I went to bed at 10 p.m. My partner said I looked spaced out. My eyes feel a bit grainy.
Evening - Eyes have felt sore today, and a friend said I looked tired and my eyes looked funny (Day 20).

4) When I woke up my eyes felt like they were 'little slits' and they stayed that way all day. My eyes felt really tired, and I felt tired all day (Day 8).

Rubrics

Shoulders

2) I realised I had no shoulder tension or pain – none of my usual pains. This also showed up in the Reflexology point that relates to shoulders (Day 2).
My shoulder pain returned, and the shoulder reflex in my foot was painful again on both sides (Day 3).
Prover's note four months later - The neck and shoulder pain and tension, along with the associated foot reflex pain, has cleared completely since the proving. Before it was always painful when I walked. *She remains clear of this symptom five years later (2009).*

Rubrics

Extremities

1) *Forty minutes after the first tablet* - I got a sudden pain in the front of my right shinbone, lasting for about a minute, then it went. It came on when I was driving, and feels like a small area is being pressed really hard, causing the pain (Day 1).
When I woke in the night I was aware of aching in my right ankle, which I broke five years ago. It hasn't ached like that for three or four years (Day 7).
My right ankle aches, slightly, but not the same as in the night.
My first and middle fingers on the left hand feel numb at the ends. My finger nails are awful – all splitting and dry. The

thumbs and forefingers are especially bad, with the nail coming off in layers. I can't seem to file them right to stop them snagging (Day 8).

2) My chilblains appear to have vanished. There is no pain, and no itching and the inflammation is mostly gone – no sensation at all (Day 1).
I have an intermittent feeling of warm water being poured over my feet: mostly in my right foot. This was the worst foot for chilblains. *In the evening* – Getting pins and needles in my feet, as if the feeling was coming back. The sensations were stronger where the chilblains had been. There is a slight soreness returning, but no sign of the actual chilblains (Day 2).
Feet feel very cold again. Most of the chilblains have not returned at all, only the two worst ones are slightly sore, but they're not swollen (Day 3).
Overall sensation of being quite warm. I would normally feel the cold on a Winter's day. My hands are warm and my feet are relatively warm. My chilblains have not returned (Day 4).

3) I've realised how weak and brittle my nails are, although I hadn't considered until now that this could be related to the proving. They are flaking and peeling much more than usual. I even felt the need to bite them all off a couple of days ago. I haven't bitten my nails since I was a child. It wasn't anxious nail-biting, more the fact that they irritated me, being so weak and unhealthy looking. Now I feel unhappy with how my nails look, and can't wait till they grow back. I'm very conscious of not being attractive with nails like this (Day 10).
Feet and hands feel cold, and have done for a while (Day 20).

6) In the evening I have ice-cold feet when watching TV, and going to bed. It feels like they're in ice-cold water, from half way down my leg down to my feet. They are not as cold to touch as the sensation itself, and warmed up once in bed; this happened on three successive evenings (Day 1).
Synchronicity?! I burnt my foot two hours ago – spilled a cup of boiling water over it (Day 3).

7) I developed a circle of small red spots on my right arm, above

my elbow, at 5 p.m. today (Day 12).

Spots on my arm have turned into a dry patch. The skin on my shoulders is also dry. I used to have dryness on my shoulders and arms about eighteen months ago. At that time it was much worse. It's like a BCG Heaf test mark (Day 13). *A connection with her teenage years showing up? Ed. See her review on page 77.*

Skin still dry on my shoulders (Day 16).

Prover's review - I still have dry patches on my elbows and shoulders, where I had acne on my back it has cleared, but prior to the proving I had been undergoing homoeopathic treatment for my skin, so I'm not sure if I'm still experiencing the effects of that.

9) Generalised muscle pain and weariness (Day 4).

Blotchy patches of skin on the left arm in the last twenty-four hours (Day 9).

By now a full-blown shingles attack has developed. Skin rash all the way down the outer side of my left arm. I can't raise my left arm, and every so often there is a sharp stabbing pain in that arm, as if things are starting to work again. Then the pain changes place. Also a large dull pain in the left arm, the lower half of my spine, the entire pelvic region, and both legs equally – which makes it impossible to stay in any one position. It is an incredible pain, which builds up and becomes intolerable – if I can get up and move it goes away for a while. Lying down is impossible, so I have not been able to sleep at all for the last two nights. In addition I experience painful cramps in both legs, and have to jam my legs against the wall. The cramps come on when I lie down, and when I'm walking around they can come on in the arches of my feet. My feet are the really bad cramp areas – I have fallen arches (Day 15).

10) I notice that my hands are in better condition than I would expect, considering the cold weather. I usually develop splits on my thumbs and on the tips of the fingers around the ends of the nails. Usually my hands are chapped, with open cuts, in the cold weather (Day 5).

My hands are OK, they are beginning to get dry, but better than normal (Day 6).

My hands are still fine (Day 9).

39

The skin on my hands is as soft as a baby's bottom! Not one cracked finger, and I've not even used any moisturiser (Day 13). My skin has been REALLY good. I've had one hangnail, and in the last week of cold weather there was a very slight return of the old dryness on the skin of my hands (Day 26).

Rubrics

Chapter ARMS
Herpes 87
Raised, impossible to raise 98
SHARP, PAIN 98
Chapter HANDS
Dryness 835
Roughness 852
Chapped 827
Cracked, fingers, tips of 830
Cracked, thumbs 830
Cracked skin, winter in 830
Nails, general, finger nails, exfoliation 844
Nails, general, finger nails, split nails 844
Nails, general, finger nails, dryness 844
Chapter SLEEP
Insomnia, sleeplessness, pains from, limbs 1695
Chapter FEET
Chilblains 607
Chilblains, toes 607
Cramps 611
Cramps, walking, while 611
Chapter LEGS
Cramps, legs 1126
Restlessness, legs 1153
Restlessness, legs, motion amel. 1153

New rubrics
Chapter ARMS
Sharp pain, Herpes Zoster, accompanied by 99
Chapter FEET
Water. Sensation as if, warm water were poured on them 639

Chilblains

2) *Ten hours after first tablet* - Chilblains appear to have vanished. There is no itching or sensation — the pain and inflammation has mostly gone (Day 1).

I'm getting pins and needles in my feet — the sensation is stronger where the chilblains had been. There is no sign of them, just a slight feeling of soreness returning (Day 2).

Feet feel very cold again. Most of the chilblains have not returned, only the two worst ones are slightly sore, but not swollen (Day 3).

Overall sensation of being quite warm — I would normally feel the cold on a Winter's day. My feet feel relatively warm, and the chilblains have not returned (Day 4).

Note: This prover had suffered from severe chilblains every Winter since puberty. They disappeared during the proving, and have not returned so far (2009).

Rubrics

Chapter DISEASES
Chilblains   396
Chapter FEET
Chilblains   607
Chilblains, toes   607
Feet, Tingling, prickling   637

Skin

1) *Twenty minutes after the first dose* - Prickling and itching on inside of right forearm, just below the elbow joint. I scratched the itchy spot, which is about five centimetres across. Itchiness is better for uncovering. After five minutes the itching subsides, but back of left elbow begins prickling — less so than right side. This subsides after a few minutes. Then same sensation in right ear lobe, which goes after a few minutes.

Forty five minutes later - Itching front of waist, under waistband of trousers. Face and ears and right collarbone have intermittent prickling feeling, > rubbing and uncovering. Sensation as if millions of pins are being stuck in – feels hottish but not burning. Rubbing it gives temporary relief.

An hour later - Neck is itching.

After another hour and a half - Itching behind the ears. In each part of my body where it was itchy last, it goes hot after the itching disappears.

Half an hour after that - Sole of right foot itchy under heel.

Three hours later - Feel much better. A bit of itching but much less than before. Feel more grounded, and less vague and spaced out; it's as if I've sobered up.

Twenty minutes later - Itching back again, around waistband.

Two hours after that - Itching on both calves, same pattern: small area itches.

After another hour and a half - Itching has subsided a lot (Day 1).

Outer left forearm has an itchy patch bigger than yesterday. There is no rash but I want to scratch it. The whole of my forearm down to my hand is itchy. I have some itching on the back of right foot, and back of left hand too (Day 2).

I've started to itch again – that same prickly feeling. It started on chin and is now on shoulders and left calf (Day 6).

Itchy again today, like the first day of the proving (Day 13).

4) This month I've not had cold sores or piles – I usually have them once a month (Day 15).

6) *Three hours after first tablet* - Tingling sensation all over, as if excited about something – quite sensual feeling – goose bumps – butterflies in stomach, like anticipation but for no apparent reason (Day 1).

Butterflies in stomach sensation again, with tingling (Day 2).

9) I'm beginning to have generalised muscle pain, and weariness (Day 4).

Some blotchy patches of skin have come up on my left arm in the last twenty-four hours. They feel sore, and hot, as if I had been standing in front of an electric fire for too long. My senses of smell and vision are more acute. The day before the proving began I had an hour of root-canal treatment at the dentist's. I was very tired around this time, and I knew that I had been doing too much. At first I thought my skin symptoms were the result of the dentistry – as if it had poisoned me, and when I became so weary I thought the dentistry had drained me (Day 9).

By now (Day 15) a full-blown shingles attack has developed – I've seen my GP, who confirmed the diagnosis. He is sympathetic to homoeopathy, and prescribed *Rhus. Tox. 30*, which eased some of the soreness. It's now all the way down the outer side of my left arm – from behind my left scapula, to the mount of Venus on my hand. (The rash remained only on my left arm throughout.) In some areas there are watery blisters, otherwise there is a raised, red, blotchy rash, which is not itchy. *(From taking Rhus. Tox. for his condition, his usable proving record becomes compromised.)*

I can't raise my left arm. Every so often there is a sharp stabbing pain in that arm, as if things are starting to work again. Then the pain can change place. It was like the pain I get from overexertion (playing double bass to excess).

As well as this I have stabbing pains in the top of my head. It's as if the *(affected)* nerve goes up into my left brain. As well as these acute pains there is a 'large' dull pain in the left arm, the lower half of my spine, the entire pelvic region, and in both legs equally. This pain makes it impossible to stay in any one position. It's an incredible pain, which builds up and becomes intolerable. If I can get up and move, it goes away for a while. It feels like it's reached its maximum now. Maybe it will begin to decline. Because lying down is impossible I haven't slept at all for the last two nights. During all this time the muscle pains and headaches have gradually become more and more intense. In addition I experience painful cramps in both legs. I have to jam my legs against the wall to relieve the cramps. They come on regularly when I lie down; but also when I'm walking around they can come on in the arches of my feet. My feet are the worst cramp areas. I had this years ago when I was out of energy. I have fallen arches.

Yesterday I was very sweaty, and today I feel shivery – I need the house to be very warm. The sweaty state is more uncomfortable than the chilliness. *(The switching between chill and sweating continued for two weeks in total.)* I have been washing, but there is a putrid smell that I can't seem to get rid of – its of rancid sweat or ghee.

I feel very grotty and am not enjoying eating. I have to force food down. I've been drinking lots of water, but my urine is dark yellow and smells brackish or marsh-like despite this. Despite my ongoing IBS my bowels didn't play up at all during this entire episode (Day 15).

Prover's review : When I was eight or nine years old I had chicken pox. It was in the Winter, and there was six feet *(two metres)* of snow and the doctor couldn't get to our house – it nearly killed me. It was the first of several near-death experiences. I remember an experience as if I was going into a tunnel, and ahead of me there was a red and a white lobster, fighting, and the red one won.

Since the proving began I seem to be more psychic: I 'see' things more. I feel my life might be going off in a new direction, which has something to do with male/female relationships. In the past these have caused me so much trouble, and I have given them trouble too.

Supervisor's comment: He was unable to use his left arm at all for several months, and remained very tired and debilitated for a long time. After eight months the improvement was complete.

10) I woke up with a developing small herpes sore at the apex of the sacrum – the first one for many months. It is very mild and slightly itchy. I have had severe attacks in the past, in this area, when my immune system is compromised. I relate this attack to the remedy. Normally it is due to feeling negative and run-down. But at the moment I'm happy and positive, and physically well (Day 4).

Herpes almost better, no longer itchy, but my mood is less positive. I notice that my hands are in better condition than I would expect, considering the cold weather. I usually develop splits on my thumbs and on the tips of the fingers around the ends of the nails. Usually my hands are chapped, with open cuts, in the cold weather (Day 5).

My hands are OK, they are beginning to get dry, but better than normal (Day 6).

Now I have herpes, one on the left buttock, and one on the corner of the left lower lip. They came on without warning, yet I do not have a cold, and I'm not over-stressed. They are very small, there is no burning, but slight itching on the lip in the morning, as it was starting. Otherwise, my skin is fine, which is quite re-markable, considering the severe cold weather (Day 7).

My hands are still fine. The herpes are still there, though nei-ther huge nor distressing. Now all the sites I've ever had them on are stirred up. Today my general unhappiness is more marked (Day 9).

Further herpes eruption on the left buttock (Day 12).

The skin on my hands is as soft as a baby's bottom! Not one cracked finger, and I've not even used any moisturiser (Day 13).

All the herpes is now clearing up, my skin is still good (Day 16).

My skin has been REALLY good. I've had one hangnail, and in the last week of cold weather there was a very slight return of the old dryness on the skin of my hands (Day 26).

Prover's review, three years later. Not long after the proving I had the worst ever attack of herpes. It was in the centre of my upper lip. (Before it had always been to one side.) Since then I have had no more herpes at all. Also when I had a bad cough for several months the herpes did not return: before the proving it would have. *After four years. He uses Pl.w when his hands and fingers begin to show signs of cracking, mostly with cold weather, and they clear up (2008).*

Rubrics

Chapter SKIN
Eruptions, blotches, red, elevated 1646
Vesicles, eruptions 1678
Vesicles, eruptions, watery 1679
Prickling sensation 1662
Prickling, single parts 1662
Itching 1657
Itching, wandering 1660
Itching, prickling with 1659
Itching, rubbing gently from, amel. 1659
Chapter DISEASES
Herpes Simplex 416
Herpes Simplex, back 416
Herpes Zoster, shingles 417
Herpes Zoster, shingles, neuralgic pains persisting after Herpes Zoster 417
Chapter BACK

New rubrics
Itching, undressing amel. 1676
Prickling sensation, voluptuous 1662

Cough and Throat

2) I woke up with a sore throat this morning, mostly right sided; took first tablet soon after waking.
Two and a quarter hours later - sore throat mostly gone (Day 1).
Next day - Ate light lunch and realised that I did not have my usual tension/swallowing problem. The feeling that I might choke was not there, so I felt very relaxed about eating – very unusual. At dinner still no swallowing difficulties.
9 p.m. slight sore throat returning (Day 2).
Prover's later comments: I became nervous about eating since I had whooping cough two years ago. I had a coughing fit while eating at that time and choked on the food. This in turn is perhaps a throwback to an incident when I was three years old – I fell off a boat into a river; I remember being under the boat and was taking in water. It was only by chance that a friend of my mother's, having heard the splash, moved the boat and then got me out; hence the choking association. This difficulty swallowing and fear of choking improved a lot during the proving. It is now completely clear (2007).

4) The night of Day 1 I woke up with very dry throat and ticklish cough, at about 3 a.m. Drank water.
At the end of Day 2 I went to bed at 3.30 a.m., couldn't sleep,

which is not like me. *(She is an airline steward.)* Coughing every two minutes, throat very dry and sore when coughing. Drinking water to try and help, but to no avail. Tossed and turned for one and a half hours, finally slept until 8 a.m. – woke up very hoarse, dry throat, croaky voice.

Feel fine apart from sore throat. It does not hurt unduly with liquids or solids, but hurts when coughing, < talking and < empty swallowing. Feels dry, stingy, burning, raw. Slept better, still coughing, but it did not keep me awake (Day 4).

Last night slept better, but still woke a few times with coughing – better for sipping water. Throat still dry and burning, speech is more of a problem today. My voice is very croaky, I can't be bothered to talk, it's a big effort, as it hurts. Better for hot drinks. Slightly coughing in the day today, and starting to cough up phlegm (Day 5).

Had croaky voice all day, but not really hurting (Day 6).

Throat not painful any more, just croaky (Day 8).

Yellow-green phlegm, voice feels croaky, > in daytime (Day 9).

Voice is sounding much better (Day 12).

Still have mucous cough – voice normal (Day 15).

Cough almost gone now (Day 16).

Cough only slight, with phlegm, but not troublesome (Day 20).

Rubrics

Chapter MIND
Fear, choking, of 1327
Chapter COUGHING
Tickling cough 356
Lying, general aggravates 345

New rubric
Drinking, desires water in sips 335

Chapter THROAT
Raw, pain 1831
Burning, pain 1815
Dryness 1820
Pain, coughing, on 1828
Pain, talking 1829

New rubric
Hoarseness, voice, hot drinks amel. 1117

Breathing

2) Had a panic attack at the party – very mild, but felt like I couldn't breathe – managed to keep it to myself, but couldn't eat cake I was given (Day 4).

4) During cycling and aerobics, felt breathless, which is not usual for me (Day 8).
Breathless from slight exertion (Day 9).
Voice is sounding much better; no shortness of breath today (Day 12).

Rubrics

Chapter BREATHING
Difficult, breathing, exertion after 232
Difficult breathing, exertion, least, after 232

Odours. Taste in Mouth

1) Dream: of skiing, and some kind of murder mystery in which I was the detective. Found a body under a lilo-shaped giant airbag – the person had suffocated from being in it and had been there for a few days, so the corpse smelled; I didn't smell it – just expected it to (Day 2).

3) Horrible taste in mouth, felt as if I hadn't cleaned my teeth all day. Tongue slightly furry (Day 6).
Taste in mouth: horrible fuzziness in mouth, at back of throat. Lasts all day, as if I've smoked a cigarette (Day 20).

4) Woke at midnight last night, my top and pyjama bottoms were damp – this is not so unusual as I do suffer occasionally from

night sweats; but the smell was foul. I got up and it was as if this awful smell was around me, but it wasn't me. I then took my top off and smelled my top – it was so foul it made me gag. It reminded me of the inside of the bin in my kitchen when you take the bin-bag out. Absolutely disgusting! I felt very, very dirty. Felt like I should get in the shower, but couldn't be bothered – too tired. Pyjama bottoms were damp, but they didn't smell like the top (Day 16).

6) Sensitive to noise and odour – man in petrol station in front of me just stank! When I came through the front door, my house smelled, and the dog smelled (Day 1).
Very sensitive to odours - everybody seems to be extremely smelly (Day 6).
Noticed a strong smell in the bedroom. As I had been on my own that night I thought it must have been me (Day 14).
Again smell in bedroom in the morning (Day 15).

7) My boyfriend has noticed that my breath has been slightly different over the last few days – slightly musty. But I hadn't noticed it (Day 3).

9) I have been washing, but there is a putrid smell that I can't seem to get rid of – like rancid sweat or ghee (Day 15).

11) Metallic taste in mouth, and bad breath. Also sore gums, which bled when they were pressed, for a couple of minutes – though I wasn't aware I had gingivitis (Day 1).
Metallic taste and bad breath still; gums sore and swollen, but no bleeding (Day 2).
No more bleeding gums – but still metallic taste and bad breath (Day 3).

Rubrics

Chapter MIND
Disgust, nausea, from her own effluvia, to 1315
Chapter MOUTH
Breath, odour, offensive 1424
Breath, musty 1424

New rubric
Nose, smells, odours, putrid, like rubbish bin 1524

New rubric
Taste, general, tobacco, taste as from 1854

Appetite. Foods and nausea. Thirst.

1) The only significant thing today is a reduced appetite. I didn't eat till 11 a.m., which is very unusual – usually I eat within an hour of getting up. I had light snacks at 2 p.m. and 5 p.m., and this is less than a usual day. Later that evening my appetite returned – I ate a big tea, but wasn't overindulging as much as I often do. Also I had no desire for alcohol, which is unusual for a Friday night (Day 1).
Had a sandwich for lunch, but nothing else since breakfast (Day 2).
Still not eating as much as usual, especially for a Sunday. Bowel movements are once a day, but not as regularly as usual. Normally it's two times a day – I'm eating less, I suppose (Day 4).
I feel a bit hungrier than I have done in the last few days (Day 6).
Midday report : I haven't eaten since breakfast, which is unusual (Day 10).
Prover's report: Overall during the proving I've been averse to salad, especially to cucumber, which seems to taste funny. I've wanted warm food. (Apparently cucumber has oestrogenic properties. Ed.)
Last night I went to dinner with friends, and I can't believe how much water I drank. I realised I'd eaten some very salty snacks. I drank five pints of water before I went to bed. This morning

I drank a pint of water to restore the balance. I think in the past week without realising it I've avoided salty foods. I've also noticed less of a craving for crisps and chocolate (Day 11).

2) Around midday I realised I'd not eaten for twenty-four hours, but still did not feel hungry. I had served up dinner the previous evening, but then didn't want it. So I decided I'd better have a light lunch. I've realised this time that I did not have my tension/swallowing problem. The feeling that I might choke was not there. I felt very relaxed about eating, which is very unusual for me. That evening I had some dinner, but only felt slightly hungry. The 'waterlogged-brain' feeling seemed to be fading. It was better for eating something (Day 2).
Did not feel hungry for breakfast, felt slightly nauseous, like sickness in pregnancy. Still not hungry for much lunch or dinner. I realise I have not been drinking as much as usual, and in fact am quite thirstless. I had a drink of water to rectify the situation, but this just aggravated the swimming sensations in my head (Day 3).
This morning I actually felt hungry for breakfast (Day 4).
Today I felt hungry – I had a small amount of lunch – I felt OK, and not sick. Lack of thirst – I'm only drinking water out of habit. Normally I can down two pints in one go and still feel thirsty. Although I haven't actually drunk too much, it does feels as if I've drunk too much water (Day 5).
No sick feelings – had breakfast and lunch (Day 6).
Appetite fine, no feelings of nausea (Day 7).

4) I woke in the evening with a tickly cough, which only happened when I lay down. I wanted to sip water regularly to stop the cough (Day 2).
Not as tired as normal – I didn't eat much today (Day 15).
Drank two large glasses of water in the night, which is more than usual (Day 16).
Supervisor's note: She seems to be getting a lot of satisfaction from her food. She talks a lot about food (Day 18).
Appetite still very good (Day 22).
I'm not binge or comfort-eating at the moment (Day 36).

9) I have been drinking lots of water, but despite this my urine is

dark yellow and smells brackish or marsh-like (Day 15).

10) Late at night I had a slight feeling of nausea (Day 2).
I noticed some nausea, particularly with travelling. Whereas last night it was after eating, today it comes with a slight constriction in my throat (Day 4).

Rubrics

Chapter FOOD
Appetite, general, diminished 725
Cucumber, aversion to 734
Raw food or salads, aversion to 741
Warm food, general, desires 748
Thirstless, general 747
Thirst, general 744
Thirst, general, extreme 745
Water, general, aggravates 748
Chapter STOMACH
Stomach, nausea, general 1748
Stomach, nausea, general, pregnancy during 1753
Stomach, nausea, motion on 1752
Chapter PREGNANCY
Nausea, during 1569

*Additional rubrics added as a result of cases to date
(Autumn 2008)*
Chapter DISEASES
Anorexia nervosa 385
Bulimia 390
(I consider that the Pl.w could be appropriate for such states if other characteristic features of the medicine are present. Ed.)

Temperature/1 : Heat and Perspiration

1) I think I'm slightly warmer than usual – generally I'm chilly, but on the whole (since the proving began) I've not been too bad, especially considering the very cold weather. I have noticed this particularly when I go to bed; commonly I feel very cold when first in bed (Day 8).

Interesting that last night it was warmer, although wet and windy, but I felt colder in bed, and had to wear socks. I've not been cold on the very frosty nights – this weather doesn't agree with me – I like dry and cold much more (Day 10).
Prover's comments after proving : Body temperature was gener-
ally warmer for about three weeks.

2) Within five minutes of taking first tablets I experienced energy waves and a warm sensation in my lower back. It feels as if my right foot is standing in warm water. I thought something had been spilt on the floor.
Six hours later - warm/hot feet sensations continuing . . . again it feels like I've got my foot in hot water. (My feet are usually freezing cold, and I have many chilblains.)
Report later in the day - I continued to get the warm sensation, as if someone was pouring warm water over my feet, randomly over both. On four or five occasions during the day it was like a moving wave of very warm water engulfing both feet from the floor up. On one occasion, the sensation was reversed, i.e. from ankles downwards (Day 1).
Intermittent feeling of warm water is now mostly in my right foot (this was the worst foot for chilblains). In the evening feet feel very warm – unusual (Day 2).
Went for a walk with the dog in the park; overall sensation of being quite warm. I would normally feel the cold on a Winter's day; hands are warm, feet relatively warm, and chilblains have not returned (Day 4).

3) Day one of period – felt noticeable hot flushes all day today (Day 13). *Prover is taking the contraceptive pill.*

4) Period started yesterday – felt very hot today, forearms red from heat, and sweat running down the lower back. Kept having hot flushes at work, everyone was chilly and I was boiling. I used to have hot sweats, but haven't had them for a long time (Day 10).
At midnight last night I woke up and my top and pyjama bottoms were damp (this is not so unusual, I do suffer occasionally from night sweats) and the smell was foul. The sweat hasn't stained anything, but I had to change the bedclothes, they were soaked (Day 16).

Feeling hot and flushed (Day 17).
6) I spilled a cup of boiling water over my foot (Day 3).
Synchronicity?! Compare prover no. 2's entry, above, in this section.

7) Feeling burning hot all over, and hot to the touch, a glowing heat. I feel like I want to fan myself. It's a dry heat rather than a sweaty one. My mouth is slightly dry (Day 3).

9) Yesterday I was very hot and sweaty, and today I feel very shivery and needed the house to be very warm. The sweaty state is more uncomfortable than the chilliness (Day 15).

Rubrics

Chapter FEVERS
Perspiration, with fever 712
Chapter GENERALS
Heat, flushes of 763
Chapter BACK
Perspiration, lumbar 142
Chapter PERSPIRATION
Odour, general, putrid 1548
Profuse, at night 1549

New rubrics
Chapter FEET
Water, sensation as if in, warm 639
Heat, sensation as if in warm water 616
Water, as if hot were poured on them 639

Temperature/2 : Cold

2) Feet feel very cold, but most of my chilblains have not returned (Day 2).

3) I could not sleep well, due to feeling cold, especially hands and feet, which is unusual for me (Day 8).
Feet and hands cold again (Day 20).
6) *First evening* – Ice cold feet when watching TV, and later on,

going to bed; it feels like they are in ice cold water, from half way down legs to my feet. It is not as cold to touch as the sensation itself. They warmed up once in bed. This happened three evenings in succession (Day 1).

9) Yesterday I felt very sweaty, and today I feel shivery, and need the house to be very warm. This alternation between sweating with heat, and chill, continued for two weeks. (Day 15).

Rubrics

Chapter FEET
Coldness 608
Coldness, icy, cold 609
Chapter FEVERS
Alternating, with chills 692
Chapter HANDS
Coldness, hands 828

New rubrics
Chapter FEET
Coldness, water, as though immersed in cold 609
Coldness, sensation of, though not as cold to touch 609

Menses and PMT

1) I think this weekend is a week before my period – usually I'm stroppy and pre-menstrual at this stage for about a day. No evidence of that this time (Day 4).
My period has been less painful than usual. It came on time, and in the morning (usually starts in the evening). It finished after five days, whereas usually it's seven to eight days long. Also the headaches I had from the proving were during the time of my period (Day 10).

2) Slight period pain before taking the first tablet. By mid-afternoon period pain had gone (Day 1).

4) Usually my PMT is dire by now. I'm due in three days. I'm not

so irritable with little things, such as domestic affairs (Day 6).
Period started yesterday, felt very hot today, forearms red from heat, and sweat running down the lower back. Felt weary although had had a good sleep. Kept having hot flushes at work on flight. *(She works as an airline hostess.)* Everyone was chilly and I was boiling. Previously I used to have hot sweats, but not for a long time (Day 10).
This month I've not had cold sores or piles – I usually have them once a month (Day 15).
Still not irritable with household things, and husband. Period came one week early, but was otherwise normal for me. I had no PMT. It's REALLY unusual for my period to be early (Day 36).

6) Thoughts about my general state of mind – I'm a day or two away from getting my period, usually this means quite an emotional state – very irritable, very tired, no energy, no motivation etc. However, this time I feel quite balanced. I have noticed very short-lived mood swings – feeling fed-up one minute, feeling very tired, want to sit down, exhausted . . . five minutes later I'm full of enthusiasm and energy. Generally I'm feeling quite good, fairly balanced, more open towards people, more easily ready to talk to people I don't know. More able to make an effort rather than feeling trapped inside myself, which I usually feel quite strongly when pre-menstrual. I feel more efficient, my thoughts organise easier, and I'm more focussed. I find writing essays a lot easier (Day 16).

Rubrics

Chapter FEMALE
Dysmenorrhoea 657
Menses, general, protracted 672
Chapter MIND
Irritability, menses before 1359
Chapter GENERALS
Weariness, sensation, menses, before 811
Chapter HEADACHE
Headache, menses, during   937
Chapter DISEASES
Herpes Simplex, during period 417

Chapter RECTUM
Haemorrhoids, menses, during, aggravates 1612

New rubric
Chapter FACE
Herpes Simplex, menses, during 586

Breasts

6) Slight pinching sensation in my left breast. It spread across to the centre of my chest, then back to my left breast. It was like someone pinching, but very gentle (Day 2).

7) *Prover review* - I had been experiencing some breast tenderness and soreness before the proving, which has continued and worsened. They tend to be particularly bad from mid-cycle up to my period. My breasts have grown quite a lot since the proving began (Day 45).
See also her proving conclusion on page 77.

Rubrics

Chapter BREASTS
Undeveloped p227
New rubric

Breasts, undeveloped, from grief or shock 227
(This rubric is derived from the experience
described on Page 78.)

Modalities

The word modality (dictionary definition = a form of manifestation) is used by homoeopaths to indicate a particular condition that has an effect on a state or symptom, making it better or worse. Examples follow.

1) *Prover's overall review* : Symptoms generally worse on waking, and also better for eating.

2) Waterlogged brain feeling, better for eating. Generally noticed that I was not keen on food, but if I forced myself to eat, I would feel better Day 2).

Felt better in the fresh air; definitely better outdoors, but perhaps it was because I was busy walking the dogs, and that took my mind off other things (Day 3).

In the morning I enjoyed being out in the sunshine – I feel better in the fresh air. My speech and thought are more connected and lucid when in the fresh air (Day 4).

Every day I feel a bit better, but the problems seem to start around 10 a.m. and go on to around 4 p.m. Things pick up in the evenings – my mood changes for the better, and I start to feel perkier (Day 5).

In the afternoon my feelings of anxiety all come back. I feel far too sensitive, unsure and insecure. By early evening the anxiety has eased off (Day 6).

6) *General observation* : My headaches tended to be worse from 7 p.m. onwards.

Felt fine throughout the day but fluey, tired feeling seems to come on in the evening (Day 15).

Rubrics

Chapter GENERALS
Morning aggravates   770
Food eating ameliorates 734
Evening aggravates   760
Evenings, ameliorate, in general   760
Daytime, general ameliorates   758
Chapter ENVIRONMENT
Open air, outside ameliorates 517

Sides of the body

1) *Twenty minutes after the first tablet* - Prickling and itching on inside of the right forearm, just below the elbow joint. After five minutes the itching subsides, and the back of the left elbow begins prickling. Less so than the right side, and it subsides after a few minutes. Then the same sensation in my right earlobe,

which goes off after a few minutes. Twenty minutes later I get a sudden pain on my right shin. Then a sudden feeling as if the gland in my left throat had swollen up. This subsided in a couple of minutes, but then my left ear felt slightly blocked, and a bit deaf. A little later my left fingers, particularly the first and middle fingers, feel numb at the ends (Day 1).

In general my headache is worse on the right side, and around my right eye, but it does move around. It is also better for tilting my head to the right, and pressure on my right temple (Day 9).

My headache developed this afternoon, again right-sided, behind my eyes, and affected the whole of the side of my head (Day 12).

2) Again I had the feeling of warm water being poured over my feet and ankles. This time the feeling was mostly around my right foot, which is my worst foot for chilblains (Day 2).

9) Herpes Zoster (shingles) eruptions on left side only.

Rubrics

These symptoms do not quite justify a rubric.

CHAPTER FOUR

Dreams

Here the Day number refers to dreams of the previous night. I have taken editorial licence by indicating some of the themes that crop up in the dreams. SD Ed.

1) *Putrid smells*. Dreams of skiing, and some kind of murder/ mystery, in which I was the detective. I found the body under a lilo-shaped giant airbag. The person had suffocated from being in it, and had been there for a few days, so that the corpse smelled. (I didn't smell it, I just expected it to.)

Body size. Another dream, in which I was very fat.

Tidiness. In this dream I dreamt my neighbour came over, saying the remedy I gave her didn't work, I had to retake the case and was fairly obsessed with the fact that she is tidy. In my dream that was important. Also, my house wasn't my actual house, and there were loads of other people there, so I couldn't really take her case.

Clothing and appearance. Another dream involved a woman who worked for the Body Shop, showing me lots of photos of her in terrible sequinned clothes at various events (Day 2).

Flirting. Lots of dreams – busy, loads of things going on. My brother's girlfriend refusing to get out of bed (this is quite common); people jumping off London Bridge; some good-looking man flirting with me – I can't recall any pattern (Day 3).

Precise detail. A dream of driving to Penrith (I don't know where that is) and it being much further than I'd thought. Also in the dream, a debate about apostrophes, which is the one grammatical thing I'm not good at. I felt I was on weak ground, and didn't have the confidence to argue a convincing case (Day 4).

Sexuality. Dreamed that my partner said he was bisexual, and fancied a bloke. I said I couldn't stay with him if he was going to be sleeping with other people, men or women. I also dreamed that I was in a big house somewhere, and somebody from work was eating an enormous piece of beef, that cost £39. It was very red, as though it hadn't been cooked, and he couldn't manage it all. I was trying to persuade him to work part-time, and have more time with his family, but he wouldn't listen to me (Day 5).

Flirting, and feeling attractive. Had a dream involving a successful rock star, who was flirting with me. We were attracted, but I had my partner already, and he was married to someone whose name wasn't pronounced as it was spelt. I felt flattered and attractive in the dream (Day 7).

When I woke I had been dreaming about blood – one of the girls from 'Sex and the City' told me she has AIDS, and she was bleeding (Day 9).

Related remedy. Maybe? Last night I was reading about *Nux Vomica*, and I had dreams about the positive, organised, 'knowing your place in the world' side of the remedy in particular.

Flitting between two men. In one dream I had two dates with cute men, and got in such a muddle trying to please them, and flit between them. I just made a mess of it.

Natural world and water. In another dream the Downs (hills in Sussex) had lots of woodland and cattle grids, and I was riding my bike through the woods. All the fields above Brighton were flooded, and I had to swim through one field with my bike. Then just before I woke up, I dreamt I was really shouting at my niece (she is six), because she was being so stubborn and babyish, and wouldn't do as I asked. In real life she can be irritating and like this, to a lesser degree (Day 10).

Dream of a big auditorium of people I know. I was late for a presentation, and carrying too many things – including a bottle of champagne. I was worried I would drop them, but I didn't. There were other dreams too, that I don't recall, except in one I was tipping a bottle of champagne away.

I feel different today, not sure how, maybe the remedy has worn off (Day 11).

The day after a college weekend, when we discussed the proving symptoms together –

Trussed up and attempts to escape. Had a nightmare last night. I was trying to fight and escape from baddies, James Bond style, but they caught me, and had me trussed up. I woke up quite slowly with an immobile feeling in my arms – as though they had been in the same position too long (Day 19).

Another dream about skiing and hotels, which is probably to do with all the fuss going on over our skiing holiday (Day 20).

61

2) *Nature. Trees. Pre-modern times.* A few days before the proving began I opened the package with the remedy in it, and read the instructions. That night I had an unusual dream. I lived in a house in the woods, and was visiting a neighbour's house deep in the woods. Their house was a Tudor mansion, with extensive wood cladding and beams. The huge amount of timber framework on the outside of the house was very conspicuous, and somehow seemed significant. They were having a party in their garden, and there was a medieval-type game of 'It's a Knockout' with enormous cogs, wheels, and swinging balls – all made from wood. I had to clamber through this to get to their garden. There were enormous trees, very tall and slim, surrounding their garden, and I could smell a woody, mushroomy smell. I stood at the bottom of one of the huge trees, looking up. The soil around the base of the tree was dry, sandy and gritty. I felt a slight uneasiness. Finally, I was able to leave via a five-bar gate at the side of their property, in order not to have to return though the garden, and play, or become involved in the game. I walked off into the woods. It was a beautiful place, and a very vivid dream.

Water, in pools and bowls. Left and right sides of face, make-up. The first night of the proving I had several dreams, difficult to recall except for one, but they all included references to water. I dreamt of being with my mother in a building with a large swimming pool. She had heavy make-up on the left side of her face only, none on the right. I told her that the side without make-up was better. Other dreams had bowls of water in them, and water was evaporating from dishes. I also remember a dream in which I was trying to convince people of things, but they didn't want to listen, believe me, or understand me. When I'm awake I keep seeing a tall tree, as in my pre-proving dream. I'm standing at the foot of it on dry sandy soil, looking up. It's on the edge of a wood. In the evening I kept on seeing the same tree, in my mind's eye (Day 2).

Slept well, but had horrible dreams. There were people dying of heart attacks, strangers and a friend's husband. Other people were crying.

Wrapping things in plastic. In another dream I went shopping and had to wrap everything in plastic, but the food was rotten (Day 3).

Two sides again. I dreamt about picking up a hairbrush to use. The right side still had bristles, but on the left side they had all gone. It reminded me of my dream about my mother and her make-up (Day 9).

Had another 'half and half' dream, but cannot remember any details – it was very vague (Day 10).

3) *Desperation, escape up onto the roof of a house. Succeeds through resourcefulness.* A very memorable dream – it's as if I had really lived the dream. I remember even being aware of how intense and significant to me it was whilst dreaming. In it I was being hunted down and was under threat. There was a sense of my desperation right through it. My urge was to escape, to protect myself, and to seek freedom. My captor (unknown to me) was in an unfamiliar house, and he could sense how tense, uneasy and frightened I was – and he played on this, without directly attacking me. He was definitely my 'enemy'. If I wanted to get out of there, it was down to me to pull all my strengths together – physical and mental. I had to be physically agile to get away – superhuman, as agile as Spiderman. I tried to communicate with my sister, but found I couldn't. I was quite amazed at how much I achieved by using all my resources. I managed to elevate myself away from harm, to the safety of the ceiling, and then later scrambled out of a window and on to the roof, where I had to lie in wait, very still, and very quiet – so quiet I could hear my heart beat. Recapture felt as if it was only a moment away. Nevertheless I felt very empowered once on the roof, but it used every last ounce of my energy. The end of the dream involved me noticing how the next-door neighbours were (strangely enough) all gathered on their roof, having a lovely time, enjoying a picnic, and relaxing. They were in stark contrast to how I had felt. They had not a care in the world. They were close enough for me to jump across and join them; then I felt safe, and I woke soon after (Day 8).

Prover's comment: This dream was similar to my flying dreams, in which it's never easy to get off the ground. The feeling was of having to fight through to the end.

4) Had a very vivid dream about my mother kite-surfing, and of having a vivid argument with her. I'm now remembering my dreams, although earlier in the proving I didn't (Day 28).

Sexual energy affected? I've noticed I've had no erotic dreams recently. Perhaps it was because I'm getting on better with my husband (Day 36).

6) Had a slight panic attack at around 5 a.m. I had had a dream about sharks attacking my children, and I was helpless on a boat. It was a very real feeling of fear (Day 5).
Again had a frightening dream, cannot remember what about, I just remember feeling frightened at some point (Day 6).

7) Upsetting dream last night, can't remember the details, except that it involved a shooting (Day 5).

10) *Climbing up, again.* Last night I had a long and rambling dream which included an element of fear of heights. It was about my ex-wife, and as I climbed the stairs to her flat they crumbled away at the top of the flight, and it was precipitous to cross (Day 3).

Rubrics

Chapter DREAMS
Amorous, sexual dreams 451
Difficulties 455
Escape, of 456
Fights, dreams of 457
Pursued, dreams of being 463
Pursued, dreams of being, man by a 463
Water, dreams of 468
Water, dreams, swimming in 468

New rubrics
Corpses, putrefying 454
Difficulties, overcome 455
Shopping, going, everything was wrapped in plastic, but food was rotten 465

CHAPTER FIVE

Additional Notes: Prover Number 8

This prover's text is presented here, directly from his proving diary of some sixty days. At first, when collating the other provers' accounts, I thought his experience was in some way compromised and confused by his previous, and fairly recent use of Carcinosin. So, at that time it was disregarded for collation purposes. Now, in October 2008, having a greater understanding of the territory of the medicine from our clinical experience, I begin to realise that his account is very far from being insignificant or unconnected with the proving. It stands as a clear testimony.

The first part was written by him before the proving, by way of preparation.

I notice that, when I do new things, I'm kind of good at them, at least I try at first, but then I never allow myself to become proficient. I always stop before I fail. The only thing I make a real commitment to is the Farm. *He owns and manages a farm, which his father started up.* 'The bloody farm!' I feel like saying that with a lot of anger. It's the only thing I make a commitment to – and it's my father's project, not mine. What would/ could I have become without it?

I question my sense of sloppiness around my life, not bringing total attention and quality to what I do, and the excuse is the big project – doing my father's work. It means I don't have to take responsibility for everything else in my life. I don't matter. It justifies my laziness and lack of total commitment to every moment of my life. I could be brilliant at so much, but there's such a commitment to laziness and sloppiness, justified by serving my father's dream.

I had asked him to write something of his experience of sexual relationships.

1) My mother would have liked to have a little girl. I was boy number three. I would have preferred to be a woman. I've always preferred the company of women. I've felt uncomfortable around

Males and the Macho image.

2) I was very shy around girls. My adolescence was girl free. I felt very self-conscious and unworthy about talking to girls.

3) I feel very inadequate about my sexuality and desire, and have lost my potency, I feel.

4) Sex was wrong as a child. I had to have a lot of solitary sex which is very dissatisfying.

5) The suppression of my sexuality means that I'm always fantasising and visualising. I look at women constantly as sex objects.

6) About the relationship I had with my first wife: I can't remember making love with her, although we did. She was the first person I fell in love with. I felt superior to her; she was stronger in some senses. I put her down too much. In all relationships there is a part of me that always stays safe.

I'm no good.   I'm not worth it.   I'm a failure.

I have to do it (the farm work).   I want to be loved.

I want to dedicate my life to the highest.

Intention for this time of the proving: to align my energy structure to the forces of evolution; to take this time to relax, renew, refuel enjoy each moment. It's all OK. Really make that inner connection strong. Don't be afraid to open up and share. What have you got to lose? You've already lost everything!

During the week before the proving - A dream. Dreamt of being asked to fly Concord, single handed back from the US to the UK. It worried me – I realised I didn't have enough experience for take off and landing – so didn't do it in practice!

Received the tablets. Feeling of wanting to be clear about my goals, then working systematically to achieve them. Feeling to be more organised and self-disciplined. Felt more contented and positive at work, less worried – accepting.

Another dream. Woke to a dream of being in bed with my current girlfriend, and making love to her from a sleepy state. Then realised I was making love to myself and that there was someone else there who was actually sneakily trying to have her. This opened me up to many of my past relationships: how I've been left alone, with myself; and my partner has turned to someone else. That's my fear of being betrayed. So often my relationship with someone else has been pure fantasy and I've stayed alone. So much like my Aunt who brought me up.

My whole life style and belief patterns make me be alone

and my relationships are safe ones – with God, or fantasies that I build in my head; the same feelings, even as a child, but projected on to different people. Dream relationships.

The following day. A calmer quiet day, as if something felt completed.

Next day. A muddly day – my dreams, aspirations and goals weren't achieved, by my muddly way of thinking and working.

Another dream. Woke to the dream of this big Gorilla, sad and lost in captivity being visited by all these little monkeys who were small enough to get through the security fence, who came to play with him to cheer him up.

My associations with this dream: I have received a card recently of a Pied Piper – charming all the fairies in the woodland; also, last night, Tony Blair, the Prime Minister was being quizzed by a panel of the public (about 'Top up' fees for university); also my situation, of working very hard to run my business – needing little events and incidences to cheer me up and help me along.

Dream: of my Ford Transit, broken down, parked on a corner on the wrong side of the road with my partner and her girl child in it – hit by another car on the front. Little girl OK. My partner severely injured/dead? Similar to the Gladiator film I watched last night.

Morning of taking the first tablet - Woke to a dream of my elder brother wanting to come and work for me with his Mini digger. I wondered if I wanted the hassle, but there was a little job that needed doing with a machine.

Took first tablet. Felt kind of chilly all day. I found myself more absorbed in what I was doing every moment. Less concerned about what had to be achieved. Generally felt OK about everything (Day 1).

Slept well, deeply and longer. Felt less motivated to get up and go to work. Dreamt of a Jumbo Jet crash landing in the sea off Eastbourne (East Sussex). I was with my girlfriend and her daughter on the seafront – I called the emergency services, then helped in the rescue; lots of little boats going out to ferry survivors to shore. I found evidence that I had once flown on that plane. Mostly everyone survived. One passenger who appeared dead later revived.

Today it was more difficult than usual to get into work

mode, but once I did I was quite content (Day 2).

Had a warm, deep sleep. Pleasant dream of being with my girlfriend. Woke feeling relaxed, and looked at my situation dispassionately.

A good, steady day. Not beating myself up too much about not achieving everything my mind would like to achieve – a certain amount of acceptance (Day 4).

Found it very hard to work first thing – Monday morning blues, but these cleared by 11 a.m., followed by a much more positive feeling which lasted all day (Day 5).

Slept lightly; woke up with intense pain around the anus – a pain I sometimes get after intense sex and ejaculation. It intensifies until it's almost unbearable and then it slowly dies. I feel it's somehow down to intense anxiety and inadequacy pains *(sic)* – it kept me awake for about an hour, while I don't know what to do with myself during the episode.

As a child I had an inguinal hernia. One of my testicles never dropped, so was taken out, maybe resulting in this pain.
A good positive day though I'm probably wanting too much perfection at work, too much attention to detail, so I'm not seeing the overall perspective – my usual problem (Day 6).
His supervisor (also his homoeopath) says that Carcinosin is one of his remedies.

Woke early for work having slept well, but with a sense of unease and worry – maybe because I've been putting off what I have to do (Day 7).

Woke with feelings of anxiety, related to how I get my ideas of pruning over to my staff – how to get them to think like I think! If I worry them too much, then they lose confidence and quality goes down – but if I say nothing it's still wrong. So I pray for wisdom to find the middle way; but I feel so nervous and inadequate (Day 8).
Supervisor's observation: Return of old symptoms, worsened by the proving, I suspect.

A day of anxiety and doubt – I can just about take care of myself, but taking care of others is more difficult (Day 9).

Woke with a feeling of humility and asking for strength and guidance, realising that the only desire is to desire inner peace and contentment, and that in that state everything is OK and anything is possible (Day 10).

Slept well, but still tired. Realise that my focus needs to be centred and trusting. A steady, kind of accepting day – felt that with focus everything is possible. One slight panic attack, just before midday (Day 11).

Supervisor's note: he used to get these a lot, but hadn't had them for some time.

Slept well, but not enough. Felt more positive – determined to stay that way; be clearer. A steady, calm day – a feeling of completeness and wholeness – that I'm OK no matter what people may think or judge (Day 12).

Woke realising how my life makes me feel rather solitary – how I prefer to work on my own; but maybe that's a defensive reaction – actually I prefer company, but my shyness and sense of inadequacy makes me choose the solitary life. A very mild day – realised that I must put my heart first, though generally I put duty first (Day 13).

Slept deeply. Dreamt of my separated wife. I had done what I had to do – carrying things into a hall, to set up, when she turned to me and said she loved me and needed me to take care of her (Day 14).

Slept more intermittently. Dreamt of a family reunion. I was taking care of my father; each family group was required to make a video of their own family unit. I took my father back to our home where he was searching out family relics, and appeared a lot fitter out of the wheelchair than the impression he gave. I saw how passive I become in front of him – how I allow him to have the power. I prefer the quiet backseat.

A good day. I was able to express my feelings, which made all the difference (Day 15).

Awoke after a dreamy, thinking sort of sleep. Got quite depressed and felt overtired but got out of the feeling by the evening (Day 16).

Slept well, but wanted to sleep a lot more – I just want to be loved and accepted. A good, solid day (Day 17).

Slept well and woke well. A deep sense of acceptance and contentment and wanting to serve (Day 18).

Slept well. Found a new sense of commitment inside. Woke early. Prayed for inner strength and unconditional guidance and love (Day 20).

A good positive day – accepting things as they happen. A

feeling that love is unconditional and that's OK. It's not possession and ownership (Day 21).

Slept well. Dreamt of having too many people in the house, and too much going on. Realised that if I was going to get all the Spring work done I was going to have to simplify and prioritise my life; but I felt stressed with too much to do most of the day (Day 22).

Awoke early with realisation that if I carry on with this load on my shoulders I'll make myself ill. I have to find a way of beng more balanced, and to let go of worry and anxiety. A very good day. Pub lunch with my partner, and the evening with friends. Balanced my work obsessed life; now I must remain more balanced and centred (Day 23).

Woke very early, needing to meditate and centre. A difficult morning, but finally 'begged' – a cry of the heart - to get rid of this confusion, clouded mind, pain and anguish. Able to let go around midday and found an inner calm, and the afternoon and evening went smoothly (Day 24).

A balanced, centred day (Day 25).

A day when I was able to let go of this created love affair dream that was very beautiful, but would have made life more complicated, less simple and made it less easy for me to react to life's evolving. I saw the advantage of just being with people normally, getting on with things without this huge emotional energy of attachment – but I still need to feel the simple love in the silence of being. I still need to be totally fulfilled – otherwise there's a sense of emptiness that can lead to depression (Day 26).

Awoke with the feeling of being totally unloved and rejected, that no-one loved me, but practised *(meditation)* and found a more balanced place; but I am at a low point in my life, and I've been here many times before, and in some ways it seems more extreme, but also, I feel I have more resources. I want to serve the highest, but I also want to feel loved and not alone, and also to love. A good, interesting day. I let go of the desire not to be here – accepted who I am, and I want to open and share and enjoy my existence away from work; to make these days precious and grow (Day 29).

Half-way into the life coaching course I am taking part in, I am noticing my normal pattern: after the initial good act and front, once the pretence has gone, I lack confidence to open up and speak how it is, but rather hide behind a familiar lonely wall of pretence and facade. God, I'm sick of that space, but somehow I know no other. So, it's kind of a safe space (Day 30).

A day with a lot of sharing (of individual experiences), so felt much more alive. All the talk in the group about their sexuality made me feel kind of yukky in the evening, as so much of it applied to me (Day 31).

Enjoyed the sense of liberation around the transformation (part of the week's group activities) but very aware of my sense of loneliness and inability to open up and not being able to group bond – it feels that I don't have the skills (Day 32).

Significant dream of a bird of prey hitting the window and then, for some reason, I was slicing up someone's head, cutting it like a melon, in order to feed it (Day 34).

I'm afraid my commitment to my work takes a terrible toll, of my own balanced self. But then my partner left a message and I felt so much better (Day 35).

Slept well. Dreamt of rescuing people from a ship unloading people on a sandy shore, with the urgency of an incoming tide. Association with the recent deaths at Morecombe Bay? (Day 38).
Supervisor's comment: Rescue is a familiar role for him. Perhaps dreams of this have been more frequent during the proving.

Awoke to the feeling of being on a sky scraper, adjusting aerials. Always they wanted one more – so a bigger stretch, farther up for one position, then fell off. It's around one of my workers leaving – meaning more work for me – taking on a bigger workload which becomes impossible to manage (Day 40).
Supervisor: Feelings of overwhelm seem to be more intense.

Dreamt of visiting a country house with a group of friends. They tried to include me at first, but eventually they all paired off and I felt so alone. This feels like the major theme of my life, how my work and behaviour separate me from everyone else. I see it very clearly now so vow to learn behaviour and strategy to do it differently (Day 41).

Awoke, knowing that I had to rededicate my life to the highest consciousness – that I had to let go of my attachment and attraction to my girlfriend, that she must be left to be free. I love her, so I will set her free, and turn my love back to that beauty that constantly surrounds and inspires me.
Supervisor: This is a continuing theme for him anyway.

Later that day : Fine words, but when I get low during the day, my need for a female mother figure to give me love is so strong. I know this comes from lack of mothering and nurturing as a child (Day 42).

Supervisor: I would say that it is quite typical of him to have this idealistic loving response and then to have a very different response later on, as described here. But his awareness of his needs seems more real and precise.

Awoke as so often with a sense of anxiety, loneliness and longing and so I meditate, to go beyond, to feel OK, which works, but I know there's an underlying fear of failure and worthlessness that drives me on. I know that love is the underlying reality, but my reality is fear based, on anxiety and loneliness that drives me to work so hard. When my neighbour came and read passages of Kahil Gilbran and we had such a sharing, my focus changed from me, and my so called suffering, on to the higher purpose of what it means to be Human and the Divine Nature of existence. Once my focus changed I was OK (Day 43).

Dream: The village was having a Christmas Festival and I'd agreed to sing a song, a solo song; but at the time of the event I'd lost the words, so searching everywhere. I couldn't remember the words. I asked my friends to help find them - maybe they had a copy – then spotted the guy who had sung it in the past, so I asked him to sing it instead of me. Sense of relief when he agreed. The concert had already started, so the MC had already replaced me with other performers. I had to contact her to tell her of the new arrangement.

Sense of originally agreeing to do something that I really wanted to do, but the closer it got to the performance, the more my fears and panic set in, which became overwhelming, then I find a solution that lets me off the hook; so there's immediately a sense of relief, but also a sense of failure and loss of empowerment. I'm so afraid of public speaking and exposure so I want to do it to challenge those fears, but fortunately something always manifests to save me. The Universe is very kind, but then I settle back to second best, and a sense that I'll never be good enough (Day 45).

Supervisor: Perhaps he is more aware of these issues, or they are intensified.

Slept well and long. Woke refreshed and confident that

everything will be OK. Just keep a simple focus and have trust and faith (Day 46).

Dream of feeling alienated from two close female friends and then realised how alone I make myself feel and yet I have a deep yearning to want to belong, but in everything I make myself feel separate (Day 48).

Slept badly – too much worry, neurosis and overwork. Trying to get perfection in my work overtires me and makes me feel alienated. I think of my girlfriend endlessly (Day 49).

Finally understood that, whatever happens, I have to stand on my own two feet, with my own focus and praying for strength and guidance and humility to do what is right. To make a real commitment to myself, to take care of myself, to love myself and walk straight, with God at my side (Day 51).

Woke early with more clarity, commitment and dedication – I know I'm going to try to be more focussed (Day 52).

Slept well, with a feeling that everything will be OK, just need to maintain inner focus, though there's a lot to organise this coming week (Day 54).

A difficult day – under pressure of time to get work done; so a lot of anger and stress. It feels like it's all killing me, trying to do this, and it alienates me; when all I want is to be loved and accepted.

Supervisor: He hadn't been like this about his business for some time prior to the proving. This is, however, an intermittent and familiar state of mind.

Later that day – Actually, considering everything, it kind of worked out OK (Day 57).

Still didn't sleep well; woke worrying about all these problems. Need to pray for help and guidance. Still a difficult day, internally. I had a long phone call with my girlfriend – it was kind of magical. I could see very clearly that if I don't maintain my focus on higher love, and let go of all my wants and desires – nothing works. I need to deal with my inner loneliness and let the love in and stay beloved (Day 58).

Becoming very aware of me, the angry child – the "I want it to be this way." The manipulative schemer; then the possibility of Universal, Unconditional love, where it's total surrender and service. I see my hypocrisy (Day 59).

Slept well and relaxed. Please give me strength, humility,

honesty — to accept my desires, and to try and desire to totally let go of them. An aunt died yesterday and, since recently, I have a second grand daughter — I am very aware of being part of an on going process, not just me — how life, evolution just keeps us rolling along. I have to stand back and observe the journey.

A good, confident day; balanced. Pruning with two of my workers, then spent the evening with my girlfriend and other friends (Day 60).

Supervisor's final comment: Reading through this, a lot of it is very much what I would expect to hear from him, except at times more extreme. Listening to him on the phone during this time, and seeing him, I was aware of an agitation that hadn't been around for some time; also his confidence levels were poorer. The tendency to fantasise seems more extreme, and mood swings more frequent.

He was sleeping more soundly before the proving, but this now seems to be more intermittent (and more cyclic?). He was an extremely poor sleeper prior to homoeopathic treatment. Physical tension seems to be more in his body in cycles also. At one point, as his homoeopath, I wanted to stop the action of the medicine as he was becoming increasingly distressed and a bit hysterical.

SD as Editor: Five years later, in June 2009, in the final stages of preparing this book, I met up with him to ask if there had been any marked changes in his life since the time of the proving. Our conversation confirmed for me the significance of his proving experience and how he had benefited from it. I was moved by what he told me.

This is what he said :

Since the last four or five years I feel OK. For the first time in my life I enjoy being single. I feel free to operate life in the way that works for me. In relationship I would get more and more dependent and therefore weaker. People cannot be complete in themselves so they look for it in someone else. That desperate weakness has gone out of me. The remedy has helped this.

I used to think that others would judge me for being single because, in the view of the world, that would mean that I wasn't male enough. Trying to be what others wanted me to be was always more important than finding out what I wanted to be myself.

Does this connect with your relationship with your father?

My motivation around him was his criticism. I could never be good enough, never be as good as him. He died two years ago. Now I feel I have a loving father, not a critical father: a state of grace. He 'helps' me in my work here on the farm.

Has your feeling about your work changed during these years?

Before, and up to the time of the proving, I would think – why should I try so hard, why put myself out? Why not just sell the farm as land for housing or something? If it all gets too much I will just run away. Then I saw that there was nowhere to run to.

Now it's like this – as waves of circumstances come along I can think, "This is where I stand, this is what I do and there's nowhere to go." So I am OK with the work now. As a human being I'm very fortunate, I'm very blessed. Look at this farm, what my father gave me! Having spent so many years being resentful, moody, grumpy and whingeing, I now see that it's the effort (at the work) that allows the grace to come in. I am more engaged with life rather than escaping from life. For years I used meditation as running away – I can't cope. Now I use it as giving me the strength that supports my activities in my day to day work.

Life gets more and more interesting. I feel very enriched. I don't get the black holes I used to. I am more accepting of things as they are. I have stopped fighting myself so much.

Other provers' additional notes

Additional notes from Prover no. 2

During the Proving I wrote the following notes:

I feel crushed by life; I feel life continually pushes me to be tougher than I really am. I pictured a flower naively trying to grow, crushed by something simple like the hand of a child. Every time this happens the flower picks itself up, straightens its petals, and tries to grow again. But each time it happens the crumpled petals don't smooth out so well and the flower looks a little more ragged. I think I felt I was fragile, too weak to withstand events that were occurring, although I also felt resilient enough to keep on picking myself up and trying again. I felt that events left a permanent mark on me.

During the proving I found myself watching people, wishing I was invisible. I wrote: I feel like I'm existing in an empty, grey world, as if I'm an observer of everyone else. It's like everyone else is in a plastic bubble and I am on the outside, looking in. I desperately want to be a part of this world; I want to fit in, but I am one of the disqualified. I feel sure that everyone one else is happy, except me. I wonder why this is? I am not a bad person. I feel that if I was a better person I could make things right for everyone around me, and it is my fault that things aren't so good.

I feel different from everyone else, I feel like I am made of different stuff, an outsider. This is a lonely place to be. I feel totally alone in the world, and vulnerable. Everywhere I go I feel separate from everyone else, it's like there is a void around me, a space. This space makes me feel conspicuous, but I don't want to be noticed. I don't want to be noticed for being different – the world feels like a hostile place to be in if you are different. I fear people noticing me and this makes me feel panicky - today I felt I couldn't breathe.

I feel detached and disconnected from everything I am doing; its like I am a machine. I am only able to interact with people mechanically. I can be precise and accurate if I do not involve my emotions. If I don't put myself into things, then I can do them well. I feel I'm best with my emotions closed off.

I felt as if interacting with people was a task and there was a right and a wrong way to do it. I felt that the right way was to make the experience great for them e.g. say and do the things that make them feel good. This is probably a significant trait of my character but I wouldn't normally view it so mechanically.

There seemed to be no degrees with my observations – it was all or nothing, black or white, and I didn't seem to doubt what I saw or felt.

I doubted lots of things about myself; I felt everything I did was rubbish. I felt my job was an embarrassment to my husband, and I was a bad wife, mother, friend. I felt a complete 'letdown' to everyone and especially to myself. My self-esteem was at zero.

I also noted: It occurred to me today that I have lost

weight over the last week. I feel enthusiastic about this – I feel I can control my life by being thinner. I can control what I eat and I can lose more weight, and I feel empowered by this. I feel then I will be more acceptable. I will fit in better if I'm thinner.

I am totally unable to multi-task anymore. I normally can do several things at once – read, watch TV, talk etc. – but I am finding that I can only do one thing at a time, and I'm struggling to do that. I can't follow the plot of a film, or time the cooking of a meal properly.

Now that the proving is over I find it hard to identify with what I wrote – it's almost like reading another person's notes. At the time I felt I couldn't talk about it and I tried to put on a brave face.

Proving Conclusion from Prover no. 7

During the proving I was utterly convinced that I had taken the placebo. Then, when I was told that I had been taking the 200 CH potency I was very surprised, but thought that the remedy couldn't have had much of a resonance with me as no real changes had taken place. However, at the final group discussion all kinds of extraordinary connections were made which I found unexpectedly healing.

I have always known myself to be quite guarded with my emotions, not wanting to 'put upon' other people. Although I can talk about my emotions and feelings quite easily, having gone through counselling and therapy at various stages, I find it very hard to let raw emotions out and cry or be angry. However, since the proving began I find myself much better able to express my emotions as and when I feel them, which is different from analysing my emotions after an event. This hasn't been easy, and I've been helped by an encouraging partner.

I think that all these changes are best explained with reference to my past. My mother died of cancer (originally of the breast) when I was eighteen, just days after my last A level exam, which I guess signifies the end of my teenage years. She had originally been diagnosed when I was twelve, so she battled against it for six tough years, and most of my memories of her are from those years. I had an extremely close bond with my mother, perhaps more so because of her illness, and the impending threat that put on our relationship. During that time I was a very 'good' teenager, working hard at school and not rebellious or stroppy, as a teenager is supposed to be. I didn't want to cause problems within the family, and wanted to be strong for my mother. Even when I became heavily depressed when I was sixteen, I felt as if I had no justification for feeling that way, and that I wanted to push those feelings back down. I remember being praised by family friends at my mother's memorial service, when I spoke and was so 'strong'. I felt weak when I cried, which is something I liked to do when I was alone. Looking at my teenage years, which are meant to be ones of growth and expression, I wanted to fight against my feelings.

Later, when I was twenty-one at university I became anorexic for a short time, again trying to restrict my growth. During much of this time my periods stopped, again stopping myself becoming a woman, eventually getting started again a couple of years ago (when I was twenty-three). I wonder now whether this remedy would have also helped my periods if I had taken it several years ago.

During the proving, as my breasts grew, I felt the same tenderness I had felt as a teenager, when they grew for the first time. I realise now that this has been a time for growth, completing the arrested growth of my teenage years, and allowing me to fully enter into adult life.

End of Provers' Records

Experiences of Coordinators and Supervisors,
(none of whom took the tablets.)

Supervisor of prover no. 3
Days 1 to 7: 'The positive side' – I have had a sense of having enough time and energy for tasks, as if I have been connected to, and supported by, accessing 'earth power', despite not having had a chance to meditate for five of these days. This is totally new for me, because my M.E. condition means that it is a constant struggle for me to complete ordinary tasks, and pacing myself is usually a problem. This change is like a miracle, everything feels effortless.

I have felt slightly 'wired' by juggling three meetings;

there was a room double-booked and the computer and photo-copier broke down, but I was not reduced to tears of frustration, as in previous weeks. I was almost able to laugh at it. I've organised lots of paperwork, after months of drowning in it, and a publicity event for work with great ease. I've received an unusual amount of praise and recognition, and felt clearer and more assertive about the limits of my role and responsibilities at work. I have felt connected, and not an outsider. I had three very erotic dreams this week, and one to do with my marriage breaking up. They did not feel like my dreams, it was as if a video had been slotted into my brain.

Also in the first week I found myself flirting slightly, because I felt very attractive. This was totally out of character, and sadly not maintained! My husband was suddenly very appreciative, instead of his more usual attachment to negatives. I was very pampered – he massaged my feet for the first time in twenty years.

Periods: the first started on day two and was totally out of character – it was heavy for six full days.

Day 8 onwards: 'The negative side' - I felt I was back to normal. Although I was still getting loads done everything was taking a lot of energy. Initially I managed to pace myself, but then I began to lose my ability to say "no". I began to resent the intrusion of work into home life, and resented also the demands and self-absorption of my prover. I missed appointments because of confusion about arrangements. It felt like wading through treacle!

Day 20 onwards – I started to lose whole days to sleep and bed-rest. When awake my emotions were VERY raw.

Days 27 to 40 – total relapse of M.E. Bed-bound as if drugged. On day 34 I was so depressed I had terrifying suicidal impulses. I took the remedy *Aurum*. This state had been brought on directly by overdoing it, because my judgement had been impaired by the proving during the state of euphoria and mania I experienced in the first week.

Around this time I stopped writing my journal – everything was too difficult to face up to. I changed homoeopaths.

'Cured' symptoms were:
1) Chronic tickling, dry raspy cough – this was better for three months, then it returned higher up in my chest.

2) Frozen shoulder – which I had had for eighteen months.
Also for about a month I had an aversion to wine, which tasted unpleasant.
Final comment: Three months after the proving began I still feel emotionally raw.
(Co-ordinator's comment: I wondered if subsequent taking the remedy (Plastic wrap) in various potencies, (LM?) would be beneficial for her?)

Supervisor of prover no. 4

After listening to everyone talk about the proving, it occurred to me that myself and my husband may be experiencing some symptoms . . . I have been very thirsty for water, continual sipping all day. I've had headaches that lasted about two days and wouldn't go. I keep feeling the urge to go swimming in my pool, even though it is freezing (in January). My husband is also very thirsty for water. He feels 'woozy' and has to sit down and rest his head on something. He also seems to be more sexually aroused than normal. In the last couple of weeks I have put many hours into homework and have neglected the housework and details like keeping up the provisions for the house. I have been dizzy in the morning on waking, and my blood pressure has been very low, 92/62. I had a couple of nosebleeds, (return of an old symptom) and then my blood pressure went up to 115/80. Very strange !! Today I feel able to concentrate on two things at once, both my course and the housework, and I feel better for it. My period is also a different colour than normal – it is usually bright red, but now is slightly darker, on the brownish side.

Supervisor of prover no. 7 (recorded on day 17)

This month I have been very unfocussed. It has been almost impossible to do my homework (I normally pace myself), and I just could not concentrate. I've been going clubbing at every opportunity – this is so not like me. I didn't do it when I was young, and I hate clubbing normally. I've also desired to wear 'sexy' clothes, and want to make myself more attractive – again this is not me. I normally like classic clothes. When I went clubbing I didn't find anyone I liked especially – I am looking for the 'perfect' man, not just anybody – he has to be right.

Shortly after the proving began I decided to start a detox

diet, and managed to lose ten pounds and felt great.

Three months later: I have returned to normal, I don't go out much, and I put all the weight back on, and more. I can't be bothered to look for a man, even though I've been single for four years. If it's meant to be it will happen. I eat everything now. I feel very old and fat = unattractive, but I do feel more confident and stronger.

Supervisor of Prover no. 10

On the first and second days I had a strong, pulsating sensation in the region of my third eye. On the third day I felt incredibly sexy, and wrote, 'The usual flubber felt like delicious curves; I feel conscious of all the edges of my body'. I thought my breasts were absolute 'man magnets'. !! On the fourth day I had a big peeling-off of dry skin from one of my heels, and woke up in the night to cut it off because a big piece of my heel had sprung free over the night. *(She had a previous history of cutting her feet with razor blades. See also The Cinderella connection page 184.)* For the whole of the first week I was really constipated (unusual).

On the night of the 27th January (Day 6) I had a dream of trying to move to an area where a group of people were living on or near water. They were cruelly exclusive, and refused me all help, and I was destitute until someone put me on a train to my home city. I then had a dream of being violently raped by a frenzied man, in Italy, and shouting for help. An old woman came and hit him over the head with something.

Other provers experiences
Prover no. 5, and her supervisor

This prover began to feel ill just before the proving was due to start, so she delayed taking the tablets. In fact, she was the one who was taking the placebo. Throughout the duration of the proving she continued to have health problems which were not in any way similar to the symptoms presented by the rest of the group, and was treated for these by her homoeopath.

Her supervisor, however, who was in late pregnancy at the time, noticed that her own breasts reduced in size and she returned to wearing her pre-pregnancy bra-size. She offered up this information after hearing about prover no. 7, whose mother died of breast cancer, as her own mother had also had breast cancer, but had survived. *Prover no. 7 is the one whose breasts grew since the beginning of the proving. See Page 77.* After the proving the supervisor of prover no. 5 found herself to be more affected by alcohol than before.

Notes from SD, co-ordinator and supervisor of prover no. 9

When the group met at college, for the first time after the proving began, there seemed to me to be a changed and special quality of attractiveness in the women. I associated this with the natural female attractiveness at ovulation time, since I was aware that the remedy might have oestrogenic connections.

Then on the night of Day 21 of the proving, I had the following eight, clearly remembered dreams. (I was sleeping at the time with the spare phials of the Plastic wrap remedy in the same room.)

1) I am in a street; fighting is spreading from the centre of the city. It's as if Arabs or Muslims are involved. There is the noise of gunfire coming from down the road, to my left, as if there are soldiers coming up from the centre of the city. I'm in a bar, on the right hand side of the road. On the opposite side there are (Turkish?) gunmen, shooting at the soldiers coming up the road. One of these men had a very sophisticated rifle, and was highly skilled at using it. Should I go and stop him shooting, at great risk to myself? I decided not to. As I watch, in comes a wounded man – he has pale skin, as if he's on our side. Then a large metal vehicle painted green or black came down the road from the right side, hosing down resistance with jets of water, including the gunman.

2) Intimate kissing, in a clinic-type waiting room, with a young and irresistible woman. She was speaking a foreign language, but I answered her as if I understood the gist of what she was saying. It seemed inevitable that I would make love to her, and we go into my own clinic room. Then I had an image of a big man, naked from the waist down, swinging on a bar, like a trapeze, showing his (very long) penis.

3) There was a fire in a church, on the left hand side, two thirds of the way up the red brick walls. There was a fantastic fireman with spider boots running up with his hose to put out the fire. It was as if the heat was coming out through the wall from the burning behind it. I really admired his accuracy and precision.

4) More destruction by a big fire. A building that I had been in with someone else, a male friend, was up in flames. Nearby there was a muddy, sludgy pit. Several men had been working in it, and the sludge started to suck them all in. One was going under, only his head was visible – another man came and, with a precision move with a scoop digger, got him out. Then all the men stood and were washed off with soapy water from a big hose.

5) I was in a house which I was selling to a friend. She was asking about a particular kind of bolt that was necessary to make a repair to a rickety loft area, which was like a theatre in appearance. I suggested a particular local supplier, since it was something so specialised. A group of people came in, one of them a woman who had been 'touched' by a divine experience. "I have it, right here, with me", she said. Her face was radiant, golden, especially her forehead (third eye). The others, also women, were talking of her experience, and excited by what had happened.

6) Children running a race – the first group was of pre-pubescent girls. I was playing music to accompany this event, and sharing a music stand with another man. Somehow I was sitting on his knee, or he on mine – in some way it was intimate. I thought he had the wrong piece of music on his stand – it was not what I had expected, nor did I think it matched what the female singer was singing. Then a boys race followed, and we male adults were to follow after, though I wasn't sure I had the energy for it.

7) I was down by a beach. The foreshore had red seaweed; I threw my shoes on to it, but the tide came in quickly and they started to float away, to the left, and to sink. I took off my coat, with valuables in it, and placed it safely above the water line, to be sure not to lose them, and jumped in. I had been foolish enough to put my shoes there and I wasn't going to make another error. I swam after my shoes and managed to get them, they were just visible under the water. The current was very strong, to the left, as the tide came in.

8) I was in a school playground, where two young teenagers were showing their ability to fly, on a thing like a skateboard. They managed it for a while, and then crashed into a low wall they couldn't clear, and had to stop.

On reflection these dreams seemed to illuminate aspects of male/female relationships from my male point of view.

These are some of the themes as I understand them:

Precision and exactness – tools, weapons, hoses used with exactness and precision. Also, the exact size of a bolt required for a job. My associations – the singular precision of the fertilisation process.

Water to quell fire – yin female energy cooling the yang male/fire/heat.

Right and left sides – in some of the dreams there was a movement from the right to the left side, and in many of them I was viewing the scene from the right hand side. I associate this with the top of the right side pillar of the Kabbalah Tree of Life, archetypally the male side.

Later that night, in a quiet and receptive time I had the feeling that a phial of Plastic wrap tablets was lodged in the left side of my neck, and my homoeopath was telling me to take it out. The eight dreams were enough. From then on I kept the spare phials in another room!

A concluding observation.
This was written in 2005
just after the collation was completed.

This proving may be a useful reflection of how plastics have affected us all since their invention in the 1930s, their increasingly widespread use, and their infiltration into the food chain. Add to that the mixture of contraceptive residues in our drinking water, and I wonder if male/female attitudes and behaviour have been substantially affected or put out of balance in those parts of the world that use these things a lot. If it has been seen that sperm counts are affected, and physiological abnormalities are increasing, it would not be a surprise to find that emotional and psychological positions have been affected too – particularly in respect of sexuality and sexual expression. I think that this proving can teach us something on this subject. SD

CHAPTER SIX

Materia medica, Chakras and Related Remedies.
A comparision with the remedy Polystyrene.

MATERIA MEDICA

A caution here! Remember the hanging mobile concept in the introduction; if you know someone who suffers from, for example, chilblains or binge eating, which are listed here, it does NOT necessarily mean that this remedy will be the one for them. Other typical and characteristic facets of the remedy 'picture' would need to be present to justify using it. We have to consider the whole scope and territory of the medicine, and also may need to make comparisons with other homoeopathic remedies. It is **very** *likely to be a mistake to prescribe on a single symptom out of context. Best consult a homoeopath!*

* Indicates a symptom that cleared during and that also, in some instances, remains cleared since the proving.
Bold indicates conditions or symptoms from one of the cases in which Plastic wrap has been used that improved with taking the remedy; or confirms a specific proving symptom.
Other features of this 'medical material' are extracted from the provers' records for being striking or outstanding in some way.

GENERAL FEATURES

Weight gain or loss. Body image : feels unattractive. Effects of alcohol. Sensations as if drunk. Sensations and **dreams relating to water.** Cold hands and feet/or **generally warmer.** Chilblains.* Herpes Zoster (Shingles). Herpes simplex.* Foul smelling perspiration. Binge or **comfort eating.** Bulimia or anorexia (when other symptoms agree). Feels crushed by life; **as if 'buried' or 'squashed'. Absence of joy or motivation. Looks pale and washed out. Obsessed with appearance and 'has' to use make-up. Chronic fatigue states (when other symptoms of the remedy are present).** *(See Case 16 – page 162)*

Observations from the homoeopath Mike Bridger – There appears to be a 'trapped' theme – 'trapped in a tunnel' – trapped, drowning, choking – panic attack at a party, choking. A feeling of Tubercular emotional entrapment and emotional strangulation and an inability to escape from whatever causes there are.
(For an understanding of the term 'Tubercular' see Colin Griffith's book The Companion to Homoeopathy.)

MODALITIES

Worse : morning, evening, or < daytime and > by early evening.
< Alcohol.
Better : **open air**, eating, bowel movements, **expressing thoughts and feelings.**

MIND AND EMOTIONS

Vivacity. **Talkative. Talks about herself.** Exhilarated. Enhanced perceptions. Sensitive to noise and smells. **Speaks out. Keen to clean (in the home).** Multi-tasking. Precise detail. Organised and able to concentrate well. Calmness and focus.
OR – Clumsy and cautious. **Overwhelmed, with a desire to get away, to 'escape' from the pressure of her everyday situation. Impatience. Procrastinating. Sadness. Unmotivated. Mental confusion and agitation. Panic in the supermarket.** Spaced out. Loss of sense of time. Absent-minded with difficulties concentrating.
Sense of connection or separation in relation to others. Issues to do with body image: feels unattractive, sensitive to the opinions of others (particularly about appearance). Reserved with acute feelings of embarrassment. Lack of confidence and self-esteem. Uncertainty about sexual orientation. Self-harm.

ABDOMEN Sense of anticipation, of 'butterflies'.

BREASTS Delayed development, possibly from times of emotional difficulty,* and grief?

EYES Sore and tired.

FEMALE PMT. **Irritable before period.** Painful periods. Herpes simplex during periods. **Water retention during periods.**
Symptoms in pregnancy – nausea, heartburn, carpal tunnel *(See Case 11 - page 131).*

FOOD **Appetite diminished**/Binge or **comfort eating.** Desires warm/averse raw foods, averse cucumber. Thirstless or thirsty.

HEAD **Headaches. Sense of pressure. Temples. Behind eyes. < Right side, > pressure, > leaning head to the right. Dizziness. Groggy feeling, like a hangover,** < alcohol.

LIMBS Finger nails brittle and flaking. Cracks and dryness around finger tips in the winter.* (In shingles) difficulty raising arms and painful cramps in legs.

LUNGS Breathless from exertion.

MOUTH Musty, offensive odour of breath.

SHOULDERS Pain and tension. Frozen shoulder.*

SKIN Dryness. Rough, chapped, cracked skin, especially hands.* Itching. Prickling. Tingling. Herpes simplex.*

SLEEP Dreams – of difficulties, of being pursued, of fights, **of escape. Of water.** Sexual dreams.

STOMACH Nausea < motion. **Nausea of pregnancy.**

TEMPERATURE Cold (hands and feet) or else **warmer generally.** Fever: alternation of perspiration with heat, and extreme chilliness, with shingles.

THROAT Tension. Difficulty swallowing, and fear of choking.* Dry, sore throat < coughing, talking, empty swallowing.

CHAKRAS

Third eye/Crown.   Glowing natural brightness showing around face and head after having benefited from the remedy.
Throat Singing. > Expressing feelings.
Sacral Dreams of water. Water as a central aspect, symbolically? *(I recommend the section on the sacral chakra in Naomi Ozaniec's book The Elements of the Chakras. Element Books. 1996. I quote: 'The sexual energies can be aligned to the higher centres, especially the throat centre. There is a natural polarity between the forces of these two centres . . . inner state: self confidence and well being.')*
Natural attractiveness, c.f. ovulation time.
Base Grounding. Panic states in public places.

Plastic wrap related remedies

These are remedies that have been useful to patients, either before or after experiencing benefits from Pl.w.

Carcinosin. Consider here the possible links between HRT and the risk of subsequent uterine or breast cancer. Plastics in the food chain may have hormone disrupting effects.

Sepia Staphisagria Syphilinum Natrum phosphoricum Natrum muriaticum Sea Salt Anacardium Sulphur Oak Silica Platina Conium Pulsatilla Buddleia White Chestnut

(For information about Buddleia, Oak, Sea Salt and White Chestnut see Colin Griffith's The New Materia Medica. Watkins 2007.)

Homoeopath Mike Bridger's comments from reading the proving: 'Lots of physical Sepia and Sulphur but averse people. Being looked at and yet lonely . . .   Natrum muriaticum/Pulsatilla dynamic.'

A comparison of themes, considering the proving of another oil-derived substance.

Polystyrene. This proving was directed by Dr Rajan Sankaran in 1995 with ten provers. They were given one dose each of the substance, in the 30 CH potency.

Themes . Those in italics include features in common with Plastic wrap.

1. *No feeling, no involvement. Practical. No positive, or negative feelings. No feeling of participation.*
2. *Everything should be in its place.*
3. Something expensive and delicate which has to be preserved and not used in everyday life.
4. *Dirty, disgusting feeling.*
5. *I am not going to be taken for granted. Hatred towards people who take me for granted.*
6. *"Give me my place, my respect." Well-known actress coming down to an ordinary position.*
7. *Need for too much contact with friends.*
8. Sudden change and surprise, things are happening and suddenly something else happens.
9. No embarrassment in situations of guilt and embarrassment. No feeling from threat of rape.
10. *I can't face the situation if I have fear, but only if I am brave.*
11. Emotionless, practical way. Should have the presence of mind, be sharp.
12. Person who is popular with people. Wins awards without preparation. Many degrees in various disciplines. Humble though others think he is great. Tremendous will: lost weight by eating same food for one year. Indifference to appearance. Egoless.
13. Grandmother being kept separate from others because she is of no use. One just uses others for their own benefit. Well-known actress says she was used by the film industry.
14. When one is in trouble, everyone cares for that person.
15. Money, materialistic.
16. Indolence, lack of ambition. Ambition. Desire for tough intellectual work.

These extracts from the Polystyrene proving show further areas of similarity:

Cleanliness/Order In the evenings, a desire to keep things clean and in their proper place, and to have everything in a good appearance. Desire to do a lot of cleaning in the house, which I normally postpone.

Contact/Care Needed a lot of cuddling, contact, so that I was sapping out, draining others. As if I had lost someone who was very dear. *Compare here the attention seeking of Plastic wrap. Missing mother (proving and some cases).*

Love contact, even with strangers in bus, which I usually do not like and avoid. Badly want contact with someone of my own. A tremendous desire to travel with someone very close, who would care for me.

Miscellaneous Tried to examine, out of curiosity, how sexual perversions arise in people, right from the embryonic state.

Seemed more concerned than usual about looks, appearance, especially outlining eyes.

Desire to change my look: to wear a steel chain (that I used to wear for fashion-shows in the past), and grow a moustache.

Began to listen to pop and rock music (which I have never listened to before).

Dreams No emotions. My neighbour is trying to enter while I am bathing. I tell her that she will find me in the condition I was born in. She is embarrassed and leaves. I did not feel my usual shyness or strong sense of shame. Awoke with feeling of crude sexuality without any feelings or emotions attached to it.

Recurrent dreams of weddings.

Physical Stomach, nausea throughout the day.

Rubrics Listened to, desires to be. Looks, concerned about his. Dreams, Fleeing, being pursued.

CHAPTER SEVEN

The Cases

The practical application of the homoeopathic principle.

By now we have learnt something of the scope and territory of this medicine. The information gathered from the proving is now available for practical application.

The patient comes with their symptoms, and their story. They tell of the kind of life they lead, the situation they are in. They describe their various discomforts, physical or emotional, mental or spiritual. The homoeopath decides to prescribe Plastic wrap. Why? Because the person in front of them is describing a state and symptoms which are clearly similar to the state and symptoms experienced (discovered) by the provers.

There is a match. It is not that the patient presents all the characteristics of the remedy – nor did any one prover; rather that the strong features of the patient's case are also strong features of this remedy. Herein is the similarity.

The key that fits opens the door . . .

The 'proof' ? of the proving . . .

SIXTEEN CASES

In the cases you will find reference in *italics* to other remedies that have been given, both before and after Plastic wrap.

All remedies in these cases are centesimal. This relates to how the remedies are prepared at the homoeopathic pharmacy – the succession of dilutions is 1 – 99 parts at each stage. When this is done 30 times, for example, it is known as 30 C, or 30 CH. The 1M potency referred to in the cases has gone through 1000 of these stages in preparation, the 10M 10,000, and so on. By comparison the decimal scale is 1-9 parts; 6 X or 6 D means there have been six such dilutions.

Abbreviations used :
Rx = remedy prescribed.
Dosages: bd = twice daily, typically morning and night.
tds = three times a day. ssd = single split dose, a term used if two or three doses are taken in a twenty-four hour period.
Split dose = two doses e.g. one at night and one in the morning.
5/7 = remedy taken for five consecutive days, 2/52 = for two successive weeks etc.
Amel = improved after. Aggr = got worse after.
Symptom changes: > some improvement. >> marked improvement.
< symptom got worse. << a lot worse.
+ = desires e.g. food or drink. - = averse.
R.O.S. = return of a previous symptom.
M = mother. F = father. L = left. R = right.
Plastic wrap as a remedy is abbreviated Pl.w

CASE 1

A case from Yvonne Stone,
one of the original college proving group.

Introduction and previous progress before giving Pl.w
Female aged 32. Very pretty, dark hair and eyes, small build, slim, flamboyantly dressed. Single, three children aged fifteen, three and one.

Originally treated March '05 for post viral fatigue, exhausted and at point of collapse; joints on hands, fingers, feet and toes swollen and aching. She was unsteady on her feet and too ex-hausted to talk for more than about ten minutes at a time.
She described herself as "Normally very active, energetic, even hyperactive, annoyingly so, I'm a perfectionist, very active and bubbly, overly enthusiastic about everything, incredibly hard working about everything, a 150% person."

Desire for order and time alone, tendency to anxiety and feeling overwhelmed.
History of depression, self harm, violent/abusive relationships.
Hayfever, and erratic periods.

Over a period of five months the she made a full recovery, returning to work and moving in with her partner.
Remedies used were:
Carcinosin 30, 200, 1M. Arsenicum album 30, 200, 1M, 10M. Allium cepa 30 and Sabadilla 30 for hayfever.

November '05 – Exhaustion. She seems more tired lately and a little tense. "I've started to feel exhausted again, my temporary contract at work finished. I felt very sad to leave, I want to be with people, see friends, socialise. I feel frightened of everything, the future, failure; noises make me jump, my own shadow! I'm worrying about people a lot too, friends, family, loved ones."
Periods – erratic again, duration and frequency.
Very thirsty – water and Pepsi.
Phosphorus 30, 200, 1M

June '06 - Anxiety and panic. She is clearly anxious, her breathing is quick and short, she finds it hard to sustain any eye contact; she seems restless and reluctant to talk.
"I've resigned from my job, I can't face the pressure anymore, I've been putting pressure on myself to do so much, whatever I do it's not good enough, well for me anyway.
I don't want to be around people, I've had anxiety attacks in the supermarket, I suddenly felt convinced that everyone was staring at me, they were all looking at me like I was weird, things went blurry and my breathing was affected. I needed to hide in the alcohol aisle until I could get out. I just left my basket and got out.
My partner went away and I felt totally dependant on him, I wanted him to sort everything out, all the things that had gone wrong, I just couldn't manage. Apart from being with him I want to be alone.
I went to a wedding and felt totally overwhelmed; I couldn't really face it. I didn't want to dress up and draw attention to myself, I just wanted to be invisible, anonymous and get through

the day. In the evening I had a glass of wine and I just wanted to dance and dance, they couldn't get me off the dance floor.

I feel better in places where I am anonymous, almost invisible and just an observer; London is good for that.

I've been working very hard on my book, writing thousands of words each week, worrying that it's not good enough; I'm worrying when I not doing it that I should be.

I get very angry with myself – I can't bear it when I feel that I'm not good enough, or when I mess things up. Whatever I do it never feels good enough, that's when I have to hurt myself; it's a kind of release.

I have been feeling really angry with my ex-partner, I can't say anything to him, even though he drives me mad, I haven't got the guts to stand up to him, I've been fuming with him but would never show it – I would just be nice about it. I don't feel I can confront him."

Thirsty – drinking lots and lots of water and Pepsi, feeling constantly de-hydrated.

Digestion – slow and inactive, constipation (which is unusual).

(No return of original joint pain.)

Plastic wrap 30, three tablets in 24 hours.

August '06 She seems brighter, less tense and more keen to interact.

"I've been away on holiday and didn't feel too anxious, maybe a bit on the plane; being away was great: I left everything (troubles) behind.

I had a panic attack on the beach, there was nowhere to hide, to be invisible; I felt very visible.

Since being back I have had a chance to spend some time with my Mum; it was lovely. I was low when she left to go back to Australia - I miss her. I haven't spent much time with her since my teens when she and Dad divorced, and she has lived abroad now for thirteen years."

She talked a little about her parents' divorce, it appears that it was a very traumatic time for her, the result of the divorce was that both her parents moved abroad leaving her here. It seems both Mum and Dad are very busy with their own lives and have little time for her; she seems sad about this and maybe even craves their attention. I sense the relationship with her mother has been strained at times; on the other hand she appears to be very fond of her father who has re-married and seems pre-occupied with himself.

"I have tackled some really big things – made some real achievements, I have sorted out my car and got it back on the road. But more importantly I have stood up to my ex-partner, I have put things with a solicitor and no longer have to speak to him. I feel relaxed and relieved.

I still can't face the supermarket, I've been to busy places and I haven't liked it so I've been avoiding them. I've found myself walking miles out of my way in order to use quiet streets, I don't want to be seen. I know I'm drawing attention to myself and I think people are staring at me. Generally I like only to be with people I am close to or alone."

She is still unsure about work, and has no job, but "strangely, I'm not feeling too pressured or stressed."

There has been one instance of self harm since the last appointment, triggered by a row with her ex-partner.

Energy up and down, low mid afternoon.

Digestion - changeable, can be OK or slow.

Plastic wrap 200, three tablets in 24 hours.

November '06 She seems bright and cheerful.

"I've got a job! I'm feeling good about life, I'm enjoying being with people, feeling really enthusiastic about life, I'm really enjoying my job and working very hard.

The anxiety is getting much better, mostly now I only get it about trying to achieve perfection. I still want to be better at things, I drive myself very hard, my natural feeling is that I'm not good enough, but I haven't felt so down on myself all the time, so I feel like that it is getting better.

Things with my ex-partner have improved – for the first time ever I think he actually respects me, I have the upper hand and he has to creep to me now!

I'm not worrying too much, I feel like I've pushed my worries to one side."

Appetite good and digestion much improved.

Still drinking lots of water.

Plastic wrap 200 x 3 as before.

January '07 "Anxiety has gone, life is great – I'm getting married, work is brilliant, I love it, no stress, I'm just enjoying living."
She has continued with homoeopathic treatment and to date there has been no return of the anxiety and panic. She is now married and has returned to her previous career, which she gave up in June '06.

This prover's patient presented some symptoms that were similar to her own experience of the proving. (Ed)

CASE 2
from Lindsey Farquharson

18.04.08 This is the case of a girl of six years of age. Her parents are separated and she lives with her mother and stays regularly with her father. She plays intently with dolls in the consultation and answers questions obediently. She is dressed all in pink.
She presents with a nervous cough.
Her mother reports that she is very responsible and often asks if she is alright. She is very sensitive to being shouted at and tries very hard to do everything right.
She has had eczema from age six months, which is itchy with dry red patches. It is better now but she still has dry skin.
She likes cold drinks, ice and lemons. Generally her appetite is not good and she is thin.
Her sleep was poor as a baby but is better now although she is fearful at night and wakes with bad dreams.
Carcinosin 30

30.05.08 After the remedy she was uncharacteristically mischievous but seemed more relaxed.
Getting to sleep is more difficult but the cough seems better. Appetite is still poor.
Silica 30

22.09.08 She is having trouble getting to sleep. She thinks about bad things when she closes her eyes, like wolves or imaginary things. She is rude to her mother and stepfather and wants to be with her father all the time. She has power struggles with her

mother. Her mother reports that she is obsessed with what she looks like and says she is ugly. It is painful to watch, says her mother. She wants high heels and skinny jeans and hair straighteners. This has been worse since the birth of her brother.
Her eczema has returned on the back of her knees. Her appetite is poor.
Plastic wrap 30

03.11.08 Since the remedy she is happier and more talkative.
Still takes a long time to go to sleep but appetite is much better and she enjoys her food now. Skin is better.
She still gets upset about her hair not looking right and is abusive of herself if she is tired or anxious.
She had a dream where she was swimming with her mother over a bridge and she went the wrong way and her mother called her back.
Plastic wrap 200

30.01.09 Mood swings from 'perfect mode' when she is very helpful and tidy, polite and kind in the extreme, to screaming at her mother.
Not able to get to sleep and has a fear of bad dreams.
Not much appetite. She is less bothered about her clothes and her looks.
She is enjoying acting, singing and dancing at school.
She still has a barking cough.
Carcinosin 200

09.03.09 Sleep is better. Less scared, seems more relaxed. She has become critical of herself and of her mother's appearance again. She sees other people who she thinks are pretty and wants to be like them.
Her appetite is good and she is enjoying her food.
Moods are less volatile. Cough is better.
Plastic wrap 200

The next day she was very tearful and did not want to go to school. Since then she is not so critical of herself or her mother. If her mother says, "You are pretty" she says, "I know".

CASE 3
L.F.

05.03.07 This is the case of a woman of 41 who came to me after having a panic attack. She said that she felt abandoned and lacked trust in relationships in which she felt exposed and vulnerable. She is of mixed race parentage and was adopted by white parents.

She is the mother of two children and is separated from their father. She has a poor relationship with her adopted parents who she feels she does not fit with. Her adopted mother is restricting and dominating. She held her birth mother on a pedestal when she was a child but when she found her and visited she was faced with brutal and racist treatment from her.

She reports a dark mood with a history of self-harm, and difficulty getting to sleep because of a fearful state. She often has dreams of water.

White chestnut 1M

30.03.07 On returning she reports that she is standing up for herself more around her adopted mother. She has a right shoulder pain.

Arnica/Buddleia/Syphilinum 200

30.04.07 Her mood has lifted but she is still anxious. The terror on going to sleep is >>, but the quality of sleep is poor.

Plastic wrap 30 weekly for four weeks.

08.06.07 She had a headache for a week which was a return of an old symptom she had had when she was eighteen years old. The headache was >> dancing. She felt more resilient and robust and in touch with reality. She felt groggy in her head with a tight solar plexus. She'd had a urinary tract infection after feeling jealous in her relationship. In her dreams she had handled problems in her relationship in a different way and was not so withdrawn.

Staphisagria 200

20.07.07 She had been thinking about her birth mother and how

she had never bonded with her, even in the womb, and that there is a void in the place of her real father. She feels she is on the treadmill of life and hates household routine.
White chestnut 1M

Reports back feeling inspired and positive but with a lot of tension and a migraine. There has been jealousy and disappointment in her relationship.
Sleep was > but now is < again.
Plastic wrap 30 weekly 4/52.

12.10.07 Now feeling better about her relationship as emotions came to the surface. She is more realistic about what is possible and that is empowering. Her heart is more open.
She has a sensation as if her body will float apart.
She is still thinking about her real father and that "he is a coward" and it is better not to meet him, but also that she wants to meet him.
She is still anxious on going to sleep and takes a long time to get off to sleep.
Right shoulder pain has returned.
Buddleia 30

07.12.08 Feels better about her work. Shoulder is still sore. Not thinking about her father now. Relationship with her adopted parents has improved and she feels more supported by them. Sleep is better.
Sulphur 30

08.02.08 At the next visit she was tearful and on the verge of panic. This was about changes in plans with her partner which she found frustrating and that she resented. She felt grief at the complications of living with split families. Her confidence in her own mothering was low and she was having a difficult time with her parents. She can't make sense of the cruelty of her mother in relation to one of her own children.
Buddleia 200

11.04.08 She now reports problems with her children's father. She is terrified by his anger and wants his approval. She feels

99

her children gang up against her.

Generally she feels more in the present and no longer escapes to her secret world. There is not so much resentment with her mother and father but she is still in an anxious state. Shoulder pain is better.
Buddleia 200

13.06.08 Feels powerless over the situation in her relationship; when she was separated from her mother after birth she was powerless. She feels out of control and unworthy of real love so she cuts off emotionally.
Right sided pain and tension. Sleep is good.
Sea salt 200

07.07.08 Relationship difficult with feelings of lack of respect. Nerves on edge. Headache and nausea.
Staphisagria 200

01.08.08 At the next visit the relationship was better. She associates the right sided pain with a need to nurture herself. As a child she had hurt herself in order to get to sleep and now she isolates herself instead. She says "I was adopted by the wicked step-mother" who was not on her side as a mother or a woman.
Plastic wrap 30

12.09.08 On returning she reports feeling stronger emotionally after the remedy and less affected by her mother. She had had a big row with her about the mother's relationship with one of her children and got very angry and shouted, then shut down communication with her. It felt good not to be thinking about her. She realised that she is searching for a mother figure.
Difficulties in her relationship were being worked out more easily and she felt less powerless about it. She was less shut off emotionally.
There is no longer a sense of self harming or destruction and this is a significant change for her.
She had a dream of being free of household chores and another of being in nature on a strip of land surrounded by a rough sea.
Shoulder pain was better at first and worse again now.
Plastic wrap 30
14.11.08 At the next visit she said that she was no longer able to

cut off from her emotions but had to face them. Waking at four or five a.m. and unable to get back to sleep. Her energy fluctuates and she felt very miserable before her period. She took another *Plastic wrap 30* and was better afterwards.

Her relationship with her adopted mother has improved, as she is more accepting of how it is and does not feel so wounded. Sadness has come up about not being wanted by her birth mother and she feels very alone and empty. She no longer has urges to self-harm.
Plastic wrap 30

13.02.09 At this point she separated from her partner and repeated the Plastic wrap as needed for anxiety or despair and it helped her to feel less 'emotional' and more even.

Her period was less protracted with no PMT.

Her skin on her face has come up in small spots and is flaky.

She had dreams of mutilated bodies which she had had in the past.

She repeated the Plastic wrap 30 but as the effect became short lived we increased the potency to 200 and it continued to help with anxiety and self esteem.

Her skin continued to be spotty and she had catarrh remaining after a cold. Also sluggish bowels.
Lycopodium 200

23.03.09 Sleep was much better and she had some good contact with her adopted mother in which she accepted her support. Skin was not any better.

She had continued to take *Plastic wrap 30* when she was anxious and it helped her to stay grounded.
Plastic wrap 200

She reports that her sense of self worth is better in general and that her sleep is fine. The anxiety she feels is 60-80% better than it was before she had the Plastic wrap remedy. Her relationship with her adopted mother continues to be better than it used to be.

Her menstrual flow is better and the cycle closer to twenty eight days with no PMT. The skin on her face is still a problem.

CASE 4
L.F.

This is the case of a woman of 54 who presented saying that she felt she was 'not supported by her body'. She had felt like this for a few years now. She was anxious and very irritable with colleagues at work, which was not like her, and she felt guilty about this.

She had suffered a lot of grief when her son left home last year and cries at sad things on the TV. She had been unhappy in her marriage, during which her husband had been unfaithful to her, and which had ended some years before.

Physically she was overweight with painful oedema of the legs and a swollen right ankle. Her legs felt weak and were restless at night. She got very hot and usually arrived sweating profusely after a walk up the hill. Constipation was another problem as she ate the wrong foods, which she used as a distraction. There was an extensive list of physical problems, which she related to me in detail.

She did not have periods as a Marina coil had been fitted and she was happy with this, as she had always wanted to hide her periods.

She was given *Arsenicum album* in ascending potencies over the next few months and most of the symptoms she presented with cleared. This was followed by *Lycopodium*, which seemed to help the few things that remained.

Now and then she would refer to her weight and her relationship with this problem, which was sometimes positive, but often something she felt she could not deal with. It was something that her mother and sister also suffered with and was not dealt with well in the family. She felt she was alone with the problem and always had been. She would eat until her stomach hurt and snack all day. She was 'disgusted' by this and looked 'hideous' to herself. She would eat if bored. Food replaced safety and comfort to her.

She was given *Sulphur* for the problem of overheating and sweating, and *Lac humanum 6x daily*. The sweating improved but her relationship to food remained the same.

She was then given *Plastic wrap 30, daily, which she took for three weeks.* At the next appointment she reported feeling much better. She was only eating when she was hungry and had joined weight watchers and lost two pounds. There was a new sense of being in control of her weight problem.

She was given *Plastic wrap 30* to hold and use as necessary. She continued to lose weight and even if she strayed from her diet did not beat herself up about it anymore.

CASE 5
L.F.

Woman Aged 33

20.02.06 She presents with eczema on her hands and around the mouth, < before her period. It is red, raw, sore and very itchy with small deep cracks. Her fingers are inflamed. The skin is very dry and hot. The itching is > very hot water.

She feels inadequate, has low self-esteem and can't go out and face people. There is a fear of letting people down and she thinks she is not doing enough and is powerless.

Very tearful, cries all day. Says she doesn't know how to cope; has no reserves.

She has a baby of nine months and argues with her partner over who needs to sleep more. Feels she has lost sight of who she is and what feeds her soul.

Periods were very heavy and painful mid to late teens. In her twenties her cycle was very short and then periods stopped. Investigation revealed cysts on her ovary. Period pain > since childbirth but heavy. Sore breasts with period.

Natrum muriaticum 1M

27.03.06 Eczema > *Nat mur,* then < from suppressing her emotions of disappointment and anger, because of a fear of disapproval. Relationship with husband deteriorated. She feels unsupported, humiliated and degraded.

Staphisagria 1M

08.09.06 Trial separation from husband in order to move the pattern of behaviour between them. Feelings of low self worth. Moods alternate between hyper and depressed; > alone.

Prickly heat > *Nat mur 30.*

She has thrush, which is itchy, burning with scant discharge < night,

and piles with bright red blood. Hands are sore, red and itchy.
Abdominal pain, sharp, cramping, << walking, just before ovulation, > warm bath.
Constipated with incomplete stool.
Period is draining, heavy with pain.
Sepia 30, 200, 1M in 24 hours.

09.10.06 This has been a difficult time with her husband and she has felt a panic in her chest and tight feeling in her heart. Jealousy toward her husband who is not living with her at the moment. She fears being alone at night, fear of burglars. Her sleep is poor, wakes shaking.
Eczema has flared up. Period very heavy with clotting.
Nat mur 1M

13.11.06 Hands were >>> for ten days then <. Feels that she is not good enough and lonely. As a child she felt lonely at school at times.
Period heavy and had cystitis.
Nat mur 1M

05.02.07 Eczema >>. Irregular bleeding for six weeks and sore breasts.
Relationship with husband has improved. She feels a void on the spiritual level, an empty feeling around her heart and belly. A lack of community, purpose and belonging.
Phosphorus 30

12.03.07 Eczema <<< after her daughter had an accident. Period >. Sleep >.
Nat mur 1M, Sea salt 1M a week later.

14.05.07 Hands and face <<<. Upset but can't cry. "Something I can't reach 'in the sacral centre.'" Angry with self because can't get to bottom of it. Lost sense of who I am. Creative energy and fire is stuck.
In her teens her father had put her down and she would cry and hide. Fearful of mother who was a bit of a bully. She felt she did the wrong thing around her and so was secretive. She tried to please her. Not listened to. Father adored her younger sister.

Carcinosin 30, 200 1M over three weeks and Sulphur 6 daily.
02.07.07 Initially hands >>, then she became desperate and very sensitive to others' comments. Not appreciated or looked after by husband or at work. Got very angry, violent and screaming, then hands <<<.
Carcinosin 30 single dose and Oak 12 daily.

07.09.07 Better, generally for a short time then exhausted and angry. Feeling humiliated and stupid, undermined. Walked all over.
Angry with father. He is rude and moaning. His awareness of sexuality is immature and therefore the time of puberty was difficult as he made fun of her.
Staphisagria 30 then Oak 12 daily.

15.10.07 Hands 70% >. Still bit < before period.
"I had to speak my truth, then the eczema was better." Was away with father and he was humiliating her and she told him to stop. When she returned home she was able to speak with her husband about their marriage regardless of the consequences. Her resentments were let out and the relationship has been better since.
Period : heavy flooding and sore breasts. Piles bleeding.
Some resentments with her husband remain. They argue about childcare arrangements. She feels she does not deserve time off for herself, she is not worth it. Nervous about standing up for herself.
Headache like a band around forehead < pre menstrual.
Plastic wrap 30 two each week 4/52.

19.11.07 Initial flare up of eczema on hands, which then cleared. After four weeks she was taken to hospital with a severely infected foot. This is the first time that her feet have been affected. It had come up in huge greenish yellow blisters that burst and became infected. The blisters were hard and red or whitish with fluid in them. The worst was on the left big toe. Sole of the foot is itchy and hot at night. She feels exhausted, overworked, tearful and despairing. Shaky. Her husband is being supportive.
Period was not so heavy with some clots. Breast pain >>.
Sulphur 30 every two hours for two days.

26.11.07 One week later. Very thick yellow layers of dead skin peeling off her foot. Inflammation and heat > *Sulphur*, but itch not better. She feels despairing. Prior to the outbreak she was exhausted, weepy at nothing, at beautiful things; she felt lost and outside the world. Relations with her husband have been open and good since *Pl.w.*
Psorinum 30 as needed at night for the itching.

17.12.07 Three weeks later. Feet are healing. Itch > *Psorinum.* Had itching all over her body with no rash. Nails are breaking easily.
Hands are < before period, but not so bad, and only the tips of fingers.
Had a flare up with husband but it was over quickly; he shouted at her because she was ill but he apologized the next day. Self esteem is low before period but > the rest of the time. Period not heavy but some clots. Piles >.
She has more trust around money and work.
Pl.w 30 3 in 24 hrs and Psorinum 30 as needed for the itching.

28.01.08 Five weeks later. Foot still itchy but hands much > even pre menstrual.
Nails still break easily. Hands flare up if she rows with husband but > *Pl.w 30.*
Piles bleeding. Abdomen bloated with flatulence < pre menstrual. Also breast pain < but irritability >. Some flooding with period.
Self esteem is >. Feel more centered, less wobbles.
Repeat Pl.w 30 as needed.

21.02.08 Three weeks later. Hands << and not better from taking *Pl.w 30.* Stressful time and confidence poor.
Pl.w 200 3 in 24 hours.

25.02.08 Hands come up in blisters, deep, peeling, dry, and sore. Itchy << night. Blisters burst and fear of infection.
Can't stop crying. Feel angry. Panic about money. Why am I ill again? The itch creates a fear. It is difficult around her husband and she is disappointed. No support from him and she panics that she does not do the right thing for him and he will be cross and criticise her.

Her father is also unsupportive at the moment and that is disappointing.

She has to do some exams, which make her feel she is not good enough and is judged by others.

Psorinum 30 then Oak 12 daily.

10.03.08 Three weeks later. Tense and crying everyday. Was in a situation where she felt picked on and was very angry so spoke to the women concerned but felt weak. Emotionally exhausted and not good enough.

Hands are >, still red and dry, cracked and itchy, > *Psorinum.*

Slight outbreak of eczema around mouth.

Anxious about life, home and daughter. Angry that her rent is going up, it's not fair. Has a problem with older women. Feels badly treated by them.

Felt she had failed an exam. (She had passed with a distinction.) Sense of a block in the solar plexus. Waiting for something to change. Anticipation, butterflies. Anger and tears held in.

Staphisagria 30 then Oak 12 daily.

07.04.08 Four weeks later. Feels much better. Was able to confront a situation with a woman she had grievances with. Things are >> with her husband. Period >. She was emotional before, but in a good way. No breast pain.

Hands 70% clear. Cracks in the tips and itchy in mornings, < period.

Coping with things well.

Abdomen bloated and sluggish with flatus.

Sulphur 30

Review

Alongside the other remedies Plastic wrap has helped this client to stand her ground in the face of conflicts. She has more self-respect and her relationship with her husband is less strained.

As the remedy soothes the eczema when it is aggravated after conflicts, I assume that it is helping her to resolve these issues within herself so that she does not need to express them through her skin.

Considering the severe outbreaks of eczema that have occurred after taking Pl.w, I think she is moving forward with a deep healing process with this remedy and that there is more to unfold. There have also been improvements and changes with symptoms around her periods that continue.

CASE 6
from Mary-Jane Sharratt, one of the original provers.

Pl.w given after a sequence of other remedies, and brings a change in her response to drinking alcohol.

43 year old woman; presenting complaint is chronic recurring thrush. She also has a history of depression and has used anti-depressants (but not currently). Had previously had two years off work with depression. She is married with two boys in their late teens, both living at home. The relationship with husband isn't good - she feels unsupported by him and says they spend little time doing things together. She stopped smoking previously but started again after her brother's death. Is also a frequent user of cannabis and occasionally cocaine. She drinks heavily (mainly red wine), consuming a bottle a night routinely and sometimes up to three bottles. As a child she developed arthritis when her parents divorced.

Other remedies previously given were - Natrum muriaticum, Carcinosin, Phosphorus, and Syphilinum.

Has pain in L side of chest < after drinking.

Drank and smoked too much over Xmas and took some cocaine but has decided not to drink or smoke for a month. Dreams are so vivid - "I drink to shut it out."
Nux vomica

Very irritable and grumpy with everyone. No thrush but libido is zero. No cigarettes for a month and drinking less. Says that relationship with husband has been based on drinking and smoking cannabis together, and now she's not doing that, they have no time together. Energy levels are low and feels exhausted all the

time. No crying but irritable instead.
Sepia

Still feels irritable and is drinking again and smoking some cannabis but not cigarettes.
Plastic wrap 200 weekly

After remedy didn't want alcohol and felt ill when drank it. Pain in chest only comes after drinking. Thrush is terrible, really itchy and sore.

Subsequent remedies have been Nitric acid, Kali carbonicum and Lycopodium.

CASE 7
M–J.S.

A woman aged 32. Her presenting complaint was chronic cystitis which has occurred on and off for several years. She appears very glamorous and well-dressed, with a love for all things expensive. She is rather like one of the characters from Sex and the City (and interestingly went to live in New York for a year recently). There is a lot of surface gloss, but underneath is a vulnerable woman whose mother disappeared several years ago (history of mental health problems).

The cystitis started three years prior when she was working in the recruitment industry in London. "I was burning the candle at both ends and had rather too much sex with too many people." She lives alone and is terrified of bumps (unexpected noises) in the night. She talks about 'the little people'. I ask what she is like as a driver and she replies, "Terrible – I hate driving down narrow roads as I have no spacial awareness. I have to drive a small car".
Platina 200 ssd

The cystitis cleared up after the *Platina* and she has had no bladder discomfort. Sleeping is better than usual and she is less bothered by the 'bumps' in the night. Has felt well in herself but

is suffering from headaches. She is habitually late for work but has noticed that time-keeping has been a bit better.
Platina 200 ssd

The next appointment was some months later. No cystitis symptoms at all in the intervening period but has been suffering from headaches, about three a week. Worse from lack of sleep, emotional upset or not eating. Sensation of pain from temple to temple, like a bolt.
Ignatia 30

She phoned to say that the remedy had made no difference to the headaches. I considered the character of the patient, and how the outer appearance is very different from the person underneath and decided on this basis to give *Plastic Wrap 30*.
Rx: Plastic Wrap 30 for headaches, as required.

She took two doses in the first week and the headache cleared immediately. Did not need any more in the subsequent six weeks.

Again some correspondence in these two cases with this homoeopath's own proving experience. Ed.

Nine cases from Stuart Deeks

*In these cases I have included the clients' own words, and exten-
sively. This I believe to be of value in 'fleshing out' and confirming
the proving material. You will also find themes in the cases that
show up in The Cinderella Connection.*

CASE 8

Female, 32 years old. D.O.B. 17.05.74

She has been coming to see me for two years now. She
has Raynauds Syndrome, but our main focus of exchange and
discussion has been her relationships with family members. She
is Belgian and lives and works in England. Her mother and sister
(married with two children) live in Belgium. Her relationship with
them both has not been easy. She feels, and has always felt that
whatever she does, it's never good enough in their eyes. Her parents split up during the time of the pregnancy. Her father has
lived in Australia since then, and has been very much absent all
her life.

She is the first person to whom I gave Plastic wrap. Seeing
the evident benefits, I looked back at her case notes, extracting
from her story those features that began to change after taking
the remedy.

*Although much changed for her under the influence of
this remedy, she still (2008) has a tendency to cold fingers in
the winter (Raynauds).*

So here are the relevant aspects of her story:

"I get timid around people, epecially in situations of confrontation. It's as if there's no energy for confrontation. It's a
feeling of having to be quiet to show that you are a good girl,
not enough standing up for myself.

As a child I was not allowed to get up to pee because it
would make the place dirty *(sic)*. Also my mother was obsessed
about clean taps. She is lonely and bitter, particularly about my
father leaving, and has pushed a lot of people away. I met my
father for the first time when I was twenty. He's a stranger.
During my pregnancy was their last trial to make things better.

Now I feel some anger towards him: he left us on our own.

After arguments I will go out of my way to avoid the person. I can't deal with anyone who will make my life worse. A year and a half ago I finished with my last boyfriend. The pattern was: I put myself down, not standing for what is needed. I would feel something is not right, but it would take a while to get there, and I would try to do what he wanted me to do, and in the meantime putting myself down; or I would be beating myself up, thinking I haven't done it well enough.

With my mother I can't tell her anything - she will use it against me in some way. I realise I do things well to get approval. How do I take compliments? I think it's not real, you're just saying that. Putting myself down in another way. I'm not used to listening to what I need. I'm used to pushing myself away.

How do I get to being a bit more open with people? At the first step what if I get rejected? Will it all work out? In any case with men I have felt tense about sex and get vaginitis. When I go to visit my family I cannot let my guard down; they are going to hurt me if I do. I have a craving for family, wanting my Mum to be a Mum and ask me how I am. She puts everything on me, so I close off, shut down when I'm with her. I don't listen. It's a waste of time. So I have no real contact with her or with my sister. With her I'm scared to bring things up, scared she will be judging me, feeling I will have to do it better. They don't respect me. I didn't force anything on them but they did on me. So I go into isolation and don't engage when it's difficult."

(After I had given her Syphilinum 30 she said, "I can't get rid of the feeling there is rubbish inside me: polluted things, like if I was just taking vitamin pills as food rather than fruit and veg.")

I ask why she is exhausted. "I tire myself in my head. I work very long days and even then take work home." Why? "I don't want people to look at me and say, "She hasn't done that job properly." I don't ask for help although I'm allowed to. It's like with my mother in that sense; I'd be told off. I can't move, I have to be quiet because she couldn't deal with it. She wouldn't allow anyone else to look after us for fear we might get contaminated. Mum looked after us but didn't show that she cared for us. It was all about IMPRESSION and not real. Like wanting to show off and having to perform to show that everything is well. Here in England I can feel safe. I don't have to pretend. If I go out I can come back into my own space. There, around my family, it's alien territory. They are not my allies. I always have to be strong. I have to keep my barriers up.

Everything that was ever pleasant was smashed when I came home: pleasant then caged. My mother's parents had wanted her to be a boy and her mother was not close to her. Her father died when she was thirteen. She pushes people away and then feels excluded.

With my mother and sister I have such a great hunger for visible appreciation that even if there is a little of it I don't see it. It's all to do with the family image. They are ashamed of me. I'm the black sheep. It would have been fine if I had been an engineer!

I'm always trying to get a sense of connection with them, but I do not meet their expectations. I'm looking for recognition and acceptance, and in my work too. I'm tired of having to be positive, chatty and outgoing.

When my father visited me recently it was pleasant, if superficial. As usual I was always like the good girl: never coming to conflict, but now I feel frustrated that I didn't say to him what I felt.

I just don't have family, it's an emptiness there. With my father there's no connection, and with my mother everything is all about her. But I realise I isolate myself like my mother. I'm impelled to work: to be seen to be doing something useful. I glow with making myself useful."

Then, after *Thuja 30, 200, 1M each a week apart, finishing on 04.10.05* "It feels like my spark is back. I've had a week of everything coming together in a strange way. I'm keen to start clearing clutter at home. I'm a hoarder. I want to feel bigger in the world rather than the world imposing upon me. I always had to be little and small, otherwise my mother wouldn't have been able to handle me."

17.10.05 I decided to gve her Plastic wrap as a remedy. Dosage was: Plastic wrap 12 x 1, then a week later Plastic wrap 30 night and morning, and a week after that Plastic wrap 200 night and morning.

After a month I saw her again. "I have felt good in the last four weeks and continuing to clear things out, especially

113

things connected with my last boyfriend." *(This may still be the influence of the Syphilinum and Thuja, but what follows is consistent with the themes and general territory of Pl.w.)* "I have been doing something other than work, home and TV. I have been out twice most weeks, going to the theatre and meeting up with friends. I've had some male attention. It's someone I have known for a while, he has always liked me and we've always got on. This time of meeting up I felt more open, it was more natural from the first few minutes. At first I sat on the floor and he was sitting on the sofa, as if I was putting myself down, being on a lower level. Then he came and sat on the floor with me. I liked that. It seems that we both have a need to move close to someone. It felt homely, comfortable and OK. OK to be a bit more close to someone. It's allowed, and needed and natural. I feel I'm moving on; even before meeting up with him I had the feeling that something had shifted. It is a shift around feeling bigger in the world. It's better for my ego. Before, in my last relationship, he was patronising towards me. I was less than him; in this new situation it feels equal because it works for both of us and for the same reason.

At work I have let go a bit more, I'm doing the minimum. Before it would be very important to work lots of extra time to feel OK about myself, now I feel on top of it all in a different way. At home, instead of watching TV, I get on with clearing a pile of papers; clearing out is now more important than doing work all the time."

(Could this all simply be the other previous remedies continuing to act? Subsequent repetition of Pl.w suggests that it is making a difference at this stage. The changes are congruent with her's and others' later experiences with the remedy.)

Observation: there is a completely new sense of brightness around her face and expression; light in both its meanings: glowing, and released from a heaviness. I sent her away with some more Plastic wrap 200, to take if this newly found balance began to feel threatened.

The next session was a month later.

"It's been a very exciting five weeks. So many things have happened. There has been another man as well: two guys giving me attention! After a while I realised that one was good and the other not, although for a while there was some confusion for me between the two. With one it just felt out of balance, he would insist on things like taking me to the bus when I didn't want him to. I didn't have a choice. With the other (the one I met up with first) there was more equality: he didn't make demands of me. With him I recognised a feeling of caring deep down in my belly. I still have this feeling of an equal connection with him. So it became clear to stop seeing the second man.

I've had a good weekend clearing out at home, and applied for another post within the firm I work for. This time I felt decisive easily. Two years ago, when I applied for my present job, I felt very uncertain about it all right up to the last minute.

I had a dream with my mother in it. I think this is because I've been ignoring her recently, not phoning her. I don't want to be around her negativity, I just don't want it.

For two weeks I took nothing. Since then for these three weeks it's been one a week *(Pl.w 200)*. I took it to keep the balance, both within myself and outside of myself, so that I wouldn't go out of kilter or do anything extreme: to make sure in my relationship that I could handle our conversations and the general situation well, so that it would stay comfortable and natural.

In the last few weeks I've been really hungry: even after a proper lunch I would be starving again at 4 p.m.

A dream. I was in a theatre with a big auditorium. There a was a balcony at the side with a buffet. I was hungry, I hadn't eaten. It became like a party, with long tables like at my friend's wedding. There were guys singing and teasing me. (In real life I would hide in this kind of situation.) But in some way, in this dream, I'm playing along with it and it works out really well. There was a gorgeous black woman cheering me on and others who were saying how well I was doing this piece and how funny it was. I thought, "I'm pulling it off, although I've no idea what I'm doing. I can do what fits with me and it works". Then it came to a song that everyone knew apart from me; then the chorus, and I knew it and really went for it. I was wearing glittery, silver dance shoes. Some of the people there had been at secondary school with me. Then it was raining and I felt a sadness and wondered if it would all end in tears."

Rx: Plastic wrap 200 to hold and use as required.

After a month : "After all the excitement and fun and feeling much more alive, last week was a bit flat and disappointing. I have not found motivation at work after my time off. I have felt tired and haven't begun to clear the backlog of work, and I don't care about it at the moment. In my two weeks holiday I haven't cleared any more of the things in my flat. It is still to do with my ex-boyfriend. From a letter he sent recently I am even more clear as to why the relationship ended, but I'm scared of letting him go completely as well as being scared I'm holding on. Taking the remedy helps overcoming these fears." *(She had taken it once each week.)*

"I don't see my new boyfriend very often at the moment but that may be just as well while I am going through these changes.

This relative flatness is how I was most of the time before. Maybe I'm done with all of that now? The time spent dreading my visit to my family in Belgium was shorter."

Things were different for her when she saw her mother and sister during this trip; also she realised she was feeling differently about her father.

When with her mother she realised: "I cannot do anything about what happened between you and my father." "I felt calm and quite clear about these things this time. Generally I haven't known how to get space for myself when I'm around my mother. She's too much asking for attention." *(Maybe her mother needs the same Rx ? Ed.)* "There was a particularly difficult time two years ago to do with this. I found I was able to talk with her about that time, in a different way from before.

With my sister I found myself speaking my mind directly, which was unusual, and I am finding new ways of building up a rapport with my niece."

About her father : "I was talking about fathers with my boyfriend and realised that, for the first time, I was not blaming my father for everything that happened since he left. Nor was I describing him (which is what I used to think) as a man who had simply gone off to have a good time for himself."

Since she first took this remedy she has been to a colour and image consultant. The advice was that light colours would suit her: Spring colours, yellow, green, happy colours, light beige and bright red. "I knew it was true." *She is going to clear out the dark and black part of her wardrobe.*

16.01.06 *Rx: Plastic wrap 200 to continue with as required.*

31.10.06 *Report* – "The remedy has a comforting, stabilising and harmonising effect. When I take it, I feel safe - as if there is support out there." She takes it (with benefit) when she feels very self conscious, and is putting up barriers. "Since I first took it, I feel that I have moved on from feeling all alone, that old feeling in relation to my family."

Gap of seven months.

17.05.07 Subsequent remedy : *Natrum phosphoricum 30*
27.09.07 In a new relationship. He has two teenage daughters. One acted like the 'Queen' of the household. I became like I was as a fifteen year old – excluding myself. Angry. I couldn't let it out, so I stopped listening. Communication stopped both ways, neither side dealing with confrontation.
Relationship ended. I feel better now.
27.09.07 *Rx: Pl.w 1M weekly for four weeks, then she continued taking one every ten days or so.*
12.12.07 Report: On a high for the last few weeks – doing things, being alive, being out there, needing to communicate, i.e. not keep things inside. Down moments in regard to my Mum. Very disappointed that she declined my invitation to go to a show. I don't want that bit of my mother that is in me like a poison. It shows as an arrogant, judging attitude. I need to do something more than I do at the moment with my potential for expression. I want to meet more people. I am keen on being bigger with the world. Enjoying a Ceilidh class!

CASE 9

In this case I include indications for other remedies given before and after she had Plastic wrap.

Female aged 35. D.O.B 05.08.70

History of anorexia and bulimia in early twenties. Long-term issue of coming to terms with her physicality. History of cystitis and kidney infections. Took some time to come to terms with being a mother/housewife. *Anacardium helped this.*

Her anorexia was triggered by being around dance students, in her early twenties. "It was an ideal that I couldn't live up to. My attitude to my physical body was self-condemnatory. It's as if I didn't want to be here and deal with the physicality of it."

She is hyper-mobile: her lower back gets put out easily.

Cancer and alcoholism in the family history.

Socially "I would never fit into a group of friends, I was always the third party. I was wanting to be something I can't be. I had more confidence before I was eleven."

Menarche at 16. At this time: periods scanty, long cycle and sometimes missed altogether, up to three in a row.

"In my late teens I had a lot of peculiar relationships with guys. I desperately wanted to be in a relationship. It was to do with not being the weight I wanted to be, and I got involved in this state of self-hatred in very unsatisfactory situations. I get angry at myself for having had these relationships. It came about because I wasn't being myself. Sex without love behind it."

"I always think I'm not as good as I could be. It's self-doubt, not believing in myself. As a child, it seemed to me that all princesses had long fair hair. I resented this. I wanted to shine with fame. I hated school uniform. I wanted to fit in but to be different as well. I wanted to be noticed/attractive.

I always run away from myself. What do I do if I'm not busy? When I'm doing things I feel more secure, safer.

Generally I don't like myself, what I see and what I feel. I hate the anger that I can have. I don't want to have to deal with things, I want it all taken out of my hands. When I am not happy with the way things are going, I internalise it; it's to do with not having the ideal figure."

Her self image improved to a degree with Natrum muriaticum at this stage in her treatment.

"After wine I feel bloated and irritable. I use it to numb my feelings about myself. When I have drunk wine I feel dirty inside and outside." *Syphilinum was given at this time.*

During her second pregnancy : nausea and indigestion amel. Anacardium.

Before taking this remedy she said, "There's more to me than just having another baby," and talked of "not wanting to fit the mould *(of being a mother)* completely." *Then, after the Anacardium,* "Now I'm looking forward to having the baby. I realise that having children need not shut the doors on what I want to do creatively."

At one point she had a realisation about her angry states: "It's to do with me not wanting to be born. I had this image of a black void. I felt very lost and lonely. How was I to move? to get on? Where am I going?"

From time to time she had short reoccurrence of her eating disorder, dreams relating to it and the time of its onset. Her weight would be unstable and this would cause her great concern. At one such time she said, "It's always been to do with not accepting myself and not being able to be loved unless I had a particular appearance. Otherwise I wouldn't be attractive to men."

Remedy given: Plastic wrap 30 daily for a week. On taking the first tablet during the session, she had the feeling of needing to forgive herself.

Later she described the time that followed as 'dark'. This lasted for a week. She experienced both sadness and grief with taking the remedy, wondering how it would clear.

"There was a sense of dissatisfaction with everything around me. After three days of the remedy I had a strong feeling of disgust of my own body, then it felt so important to forgive myself. It was time to clear it now. Then, meeting my children at the school playground, it felt like I had just come out from under a black cloud. I met with parents with whom I had been having quite an awkward time recently, and I felt easy and able to walk away, realising I don't want to be in that clique of people."

Then after four weeks: "I feel alive, bright and well. My sense of humour is back. There has been movement in my sacrum. It feels flexible and freed up: flowing with a sense of freedom and grace to it. Now I'm beginning to speak with my voice and become distinct as a person vis-à-vis my mother."

I ask her about her parents. "On my mother's side there is a denial of life, a downtrodden-ness, an inability to step forward; on my father's side there is a vitality, as if grabbing life."

"Now I feel stronger and clearer with my children when I'm telling them off. I get cross, but now it's with a sense of strength rather than exasperation. I don't feel buried by it and they are listening more! From a dream I have been reminded of how similar I was as a child to my two year old daughter. One morning, looking at her, I saw her as a woodland sprite, pulled out of the woods and then tamed.

Since the remedy, I feel my spirit really in my physical body, it feels connected in this way. I have felt more balanced in what I'm eating and not craving chocolate so much. I have had times of little appetite: when I would have expected to be hungry I wasn't, and generally I have felt more confident physically. Alcohol, desire reduced, now not more than one or two glasses of wine. I have noticed I want to wear blues and greens all the time. The pains in the base of my spine have shifted. I have not had my typical left side ovulation pain."

Pre-menstrual symptoms: Oppressed feelings before, for a few days, finding things dark, stressful. Irritable. Water retention, constipation.

Plastic wrap 30 to hold: to take it for PMT symptoms if they come on next time.

Report after six weeks : Had thick catarrh in throat, and dizziness. *Four weeks ago* : Took the remedy on three successive evenings, and within moments of taking it, had really strong sneezing and the catarrh cleared. Changed to clear runny mucus. Dizziness also >>.

Irritability before period also better, compared to the past two months. *(She had three nightly tablets just before this period.)* Period was painfree, easy and light for four to five days . No water retention. Mood lifting, feeling lighter and brighter about things.

No lack of appetite. Generally less anxious and more balanced. "Not driven about eating." Shortly after repeat of remedy, stiffness in sacrum, especially walking up hills.

"I feel more confident with my own voice, and not too easily swayed. More stable."

During the year that followed she had Plastic wrap 200 and 1M as well as other remedies, as follows:

Amanita rubescens : (in a proving.) Her eating 'disorder' and the issues surrounding it came up strongly. Then, a new found sense of "not any more shame of the eating issue."

Able to deal with her mother on another level; able to smooth the way rather than being niggled by her anxieties. Resentment (of children's demands) >>.

Not interested in drinking wine. Shoulders >.

Then back to Plastic wrap, this time in the 200 potency.

On taking it - Warmth in the heart area, feeling more lively, more get-up-and-go energy.

Then feeling fat again. "Chubbiness, I don't like it. I associate it with being passive vis-a-vis getting up and going into life. I want to identify more with my father: he is more vital and spiritually based."

Plastic wrap 1M weekly, and Oak 30 twice weekly, both remedies for four weeks.

"Brighter, more at ease with myself, not so much tension in the diaphragm."

Review after eight months.
By now almost a year since she first took Plastic wrap.

A month ago, struggling, everything difficult, exhausted, adrenal burn-out? Craving coffee, < alcohol, constantly hungry, unsatisfied generally. Constipated.

Took *Sulphur 1M* and felt generally better. Better from taking more care of myself, > multivitamins, >> eating meat.

About her weight : "It has been stable for six months now." *(This is since the Amanita proving and the Plastic wrap 1M and Oak 30 that followed it.)* I feel so much more comfortable within my own body. I feel I have a strong guide to know what I want to eat. I am not bothered any more about four pounds up or down. I feel clear and confident about it. There has been no bloating with my cycle."

Present symptoms : Eyes, hot and dry, mornings, bloodshot veins.

Yellowing of whites of eyes, hardening of cornea?
Back: neck and shoulders feel twisted. Holding myself too tight, holding jaw in the night, not breathing well.

Aware of childhood context of not being listened to individually. *(She is the first of four sisters.)* "My father had a huge authority about him. There was a fear of judgement. Stuttering, uncertainty of expressing myself. What I say is of no significance. The negative thought is that I am not capable. Wanting to be believed in, for a sense of the validity of what I am doing."
Latest remedy : Silica 1M split dose.

The remedy Amanita Rubescens will be the subject of the next proving book from The Well Books.

CASE 10
Central theme: of not being 'allowed' to express myself.

Female aged 28. D.O.B. 28.12.77

16.02.05 *First appointment*
High states of anxiety, panic attacks. Nervous breakdown two years ago. Poor sleep. Need to trust. "I get nervous and anxious, wanting to please, to do the best I can. It has to be perfect, or not at all. If it's not perfect it's worthless and I am worthless. At school anything below an A would be a failure. In my teens my parents went through an acrimonious divorce. My mother left and had an affair, my father tried to kill himself. I was his confidant and not to tell anyone. At first he put me on a pedestal, he even called me my mother's name. Then when bitterness set in any association with my mother became negative for him. My mother used to say that she and I were the same person; I remember this from when I was seven. I was the diplomat in the family. I still have a sense of having to put a mask on. I feel exhausted all of the time and wired up. I was violently raped five years ago. I can be either very up or very down: people won't want to know me if I'm not happy or bubbly."

Aged 14, glandular fever, ill all the time like M.E.
Aged 22, nodules on vocal cords. Operated on. "I was told I would never sing again. (I can now after a long time.)"

Craving for chocolate. Often nauseous.

Lower back ache and pains between shoulders. "In my shoulders it feels like a heavy weight, like a milkmaid's yoke."

She doesn't hold eye contact.

16.02.05 *Rx: Carcinosin 200 daily for three days, and then as required to help sleep.*

06.04.05 *Next appointment*

Changes: Sleep > on nights when she took the remedy.

"With family stuff I was more able to put it to one side. My brothers had a huge row and I just didn't get involved. I found I was standing my ground and less consumed by anger." Generally more assertive, and beginning to speak her feelings more. Acute panic states >.

With her partner: re moving in together. Fear of loss of independence and identity. Pattern: "It's better to go with the flow and let the other person have their way rather than say I want to do something. I can't say I'm unhappy. As in similar situations with my mother, there would be reprisals.

I've not had outside panics for a while. I've gone to the other extreme: no life in me, listless, no focus, and tired."

Dream. A feeling of being locked in. My boyfriend had built a den for me like a hut of boxes, and I had to stay in there, shut in. It was to do with loss of independence and sense of identity, and not being able to say what I think, as if he's doing it to me.

"My living situation is bringing up childhood issues. I'm too tired to speak up for myself, then I don't speak. There are long periods of silence and I don't know what the matter is. When I feel depressed I cut my feet; I can't not do it. I hit myself and have done since I was a child. It's stupid but there's a person in my head who I know as Mrs Fat. She would call me names: disgusting, obese, stupid, arrogant, a complete waste of space, revolting. She surfaced when I was fourteen. I had an eating disorder at the time."

Between 06.04.05 and 06.10.05 the remedies that made a difference were: Carcinosin 200 again, then Aurum 30.

06.10.05 *Issues coming to the fore and dreams indicating core themes:*

"I see sex as a violent act. I associate it with shame, humiliation and pain. About the rape, I was not allowed to complain, it was my fault. Sex involves physical and emotional pain inflicted an another person. I want to wash right away to take away the evidence.

But recently I have been able to talk to my boyfriend about it. This is a breakthrough for me, thanks to the remedies. Then one night I was not able to sleep. I lay awake for hours. Crying. I felt he was going to hurt me. He was a bully, he would be angry if I woke him. I was very frightened of him. I couldn't say or do anything, as if I was trapped in an abusive relationship. Since then things have got better with him, also with my family; I had a really nice time when I stayed there for a week. It was the first time in fifteen months. Before family visits were associated with depression, unhappiness and powerlessness. I slept well there too, sleeping away from my boyfriend.

Before in my dreams things happened and I was not able to anything about then; now in a dream of being threatened by a man with a knife, I was able to shout out and I was heard and felt supported.

Dream. I had been killed and was haunting the person who had killed me, as if trying to stop it happening, and he killed me and the haunter too. I remember saying in the dream: "I've been killed many times."

06.04.05 *Rx: Staphisagria 30. b.d. 5/7 and extras if sleep is difficult.*

Sleep > but only at first, then not >.

"Some more confidence in myself, finding activities in which I feel equal with my partner feels good for our relationship. Mentally stronger. Standing up for myself, even in arguments. I'm finding my voice and he doesn't like it! At one time I said sorry to be upsetting him but inside I was raging. Around him I feel like a peacock painted beige. When I speak out I get angry if he dismisses what I say. I feel so disgusted with my own body, I only seem able to have sex when I'm drunk, even kissing seems unclean. I'm still cutting my feet at night when it's dark."

08.12.05 *Rx: Plastic wrap 30 b.d. 5/7.*

21.12.05 *The effects of the remedy:*

"Quite good. I liked it. I had been feeling really down. Sleep is better; it was easier to get to sleep, especially while I was taking the tablets. There's been a major breakthrough in my singing, with the help of my teacher. It's to do with trust: to know that I can do it. I have been asked to sing at a friend's wedding on New Year's Eve; before this remedy I had thought of calling it off, but now I feel I have got a right to sing there and I'm proud to be doing it. I'm really happy about it.

Generally my boyfriend doesn't support me with my singing, so I hardly ever practise at home, except over the washing-up." *(She laughed when I referred to Cinderella at this point.)* "When I tried to sing my solo to him a while ago he was very critical when I ran out of breath; I felt very upset by his response. Since these tablets I've been doing more practice. Singing is so important for me, I will definitely be taking it more seriously. I'm not going to back down. I'm allowed.

Then I was so happy after my singing lesson and I could sing in front of him. He was impressed. He said, "Someone had taken over my voice." It was a real breakthrough: I was standing up for myself and so pleased that I could sing in front of him. Before he was the emperor and I was the retarded slug who can't do anything. That's how I saw it!

Before, when there was our familiar tension about household chores, I would feel inadequate and judged by him. Now, since the remedy, when he started ranting on about it, I stood up to him and said, "Do you know how that makes me feel?" He was shocked to hear it. Now I pull him up on any little bits of emotional blackmail. Before I would take it on and then resent it. I don't do that now. I am being a lot more vocal. The big thing is that we're talking about things rather than letting them fester. There are more arguments but they are getting resolved.

About my physical body, it's still a big issue, but I have made a decision to get fit. When I was a teenager I would go running at 3 a.m. in the night so as not to be seen. Now, to get fit I plan to join a gym; it's horrible but do-able. It feels within my power to do something about it. If I get fit it will go some way to feeling better about myself.

In my dark years as a teenager, singing was my one redeeming asset that would see me through. It was around the time of my parents' divorce that I lost my voice; it was as if the only candle had gone out in a dark place. My Mum left in '96 and I had the operation for the nodules on my vocal chords in '99 after an incredibly turbulent time. That was when I was told I would never sing again. My father had turned against me and my mother didn't want to see me, although she carried on seeing my brothers. We went for months on end without seeing each other.

125

Then, when I saw her for a day it would be wonderful: she would promise the world and then not deliver, and I would be devastated again. Like a complete fool I would then go back for more of the same.

I associated singing with my right to be here; with it, I was allowed to be visible. Then I lost all that when it went. I had no shield or defence any more. Singing was my only way of saying "I am a person," and this in relation especially to my mother and her saying that she and I were the same person. That had been going on since childhood, as long as I can remember. Now there is a big separation, but I am not all-consumed by it.

Also, since the last remedy, my habit of cutting my feet has reduced a lot: from daily to every three days or so."

At this point I suggested she could take one tablet of Plastic wrap 30 at those times when she was about to cut herself, and see if it helped divert her from doing this.

I told her that in the proving of this remedy someone compared their life to that of a flower that had not been allowed to grow; "That rings true to me, it applies to so much of my life".

"During this last year, *(since she had been taking remedies)* my relationship with my elder brother has transformed: before my status was lower than him; now we are equal. So everything is in a better perspective with my family: before I felt I was an outsider; now I realise that it's just my mother and one of my brothers who are the issue. They have problems with everyone.

I have also realised the correlation between my bulimia and the issues with my mother. It was around the time that I lost my voice; my vocal cords were damaged from making myself vomit. Now I'm singing openly again.

I have my shield and I'm polishing it.

Before there were many things that I felt could never be resolved, like the rape. It was all-consuming and felt overwhelming so I would try to keep it out of my mind; now I feel patient and that things can be resolved in their order - Mum will be the last thing. I do feel sad about my relationship with her, but a veil of sadness has been lifted. I wasn't invited to her place at Christmas. Before I would have been gutted. Now I have taken a step back. Why go and be hurt again?

In these last two months, instead of lamenting what I haven't got, I have begun to celebrate and build on what I have got."

A gap of just over a year

05.01.07 *Report of the past year* : Singing at the wedding on New Year's Eve (a year ago) went really well. She then decided to set up a business, singing at wedding ceremonies, despite opposition from her partner; also to find a rehearsal room since she wasn't going to be able to sing much at home.

She also sang for a wedding in August which went well. "My partner was very proud of me. I said to him I'm not just someone who needs to sing in the shower. I need to do this."

She felt generally better for about four months after the remedies of December '05. For the first time she felt that it was nice living with her partner, and she stopped cutting her feet. After a New Year's hangover she stopped drinking alcohol, and also went to the gym.

In August she was involved in a drama piece about putting masks on: make-up as one mask, and her 'happy clown' behaviour as the other layer. The piece was about what happened when you take the mask off. She felt nervous but it was liberating overall. At first she became her Mrs. Fat persona, a swamp monster hurling abuse at the person in the chair. "I was shocked at how much rage there was." Then at the end she sang, "as a way of defending myself from my demons. I was chuffed that the piece was well received."

Preparing to sing at the wedding in August her partner encouraged her to go without make-up on. "No, I need it, I said, I need my armour. I was always embarrassed about my face going red if I got hot. Then I thought that I would give it a go; I don't know anyone, so there are no expectations on me. Then panic, I realised how dependent I was on the mask. Then in the event I felt liberated; there was none of my previous worry that it would slip if I get hot."

Since the summer the relationship with her partner has been much as it was before, arguing a lot of the time. A feeling of being trapped. Depressed about it. But after Christmas ('06) there was what felt like a breakthrough: "He says that I'm assertive, and says it in a negative way. I say that it's not that I'm being assertive; what it is is that *you* like to control and be domineering. I'm just trying to redress the balance, to bring some equilibrium. You don't like your control being threatened. He said that I was right. Before I felt I was totally taken for granted. He is still very good at emotional blackmail, but now I am vocal and say that that is just strategy."

It seems to me that despite ongoing difficulties and symptoms she has 'moved on' a great deal in the twelve months gap. She had had no homoeopathy during this time.

The current and recent situations:

Insomnia, and exhausted from it. Finds it hard to fall asleep before 2.30 a.m., then wakes again between 4 and 5 a.m., or finds it really hard to wake up for work. No energy, can't get out of bed, no enthusiasm for anything. This has been especially bad in the last month. Has been drinking coffee re being so tired, and Red Bull. "It's a tussle between being hyper and panicky or in a state of inertia."

Underneath it all a feeling of "having nothing to offer, wasting my life, not living, just existing." Suicidal thoughts.
Back has been bad all year.

Recently drinking more alcohol again and on her own. Since New Year has stopped this, realising that this is how she tries to deal with her stress.

Her feet: "It is a more conscious thing now. I put socks on to prevent myself from doing it, but I feel compelled to do it. I feel crippled, paralysed by my own lack of self-belief."

However "at times I did discover self-belief rather than relying on the views or opinions of others. I have even sent off application forms for drama college. I can do it!" "I want to be able to rid myself of these shackles, this lack of self-confidence."

I ask, "Where in your body do you feel this lack of self-confidence, if anywhere particularly?" She indicates her heart area.

As well as singing more on her own she has rejoined a choir, "welcomed back!" and helping with some of the conducting. She did a concert and loved it; her partner saw that she was totally in her element, having fun.

"In my head I feel like a flower that is starved of light. One of the images I have had of myself is of a songbird with wrapping tape around its beak."

05.01.07 *Rx: Plastic wrap 30 given during the session.*
Reactions during the following ten minutes –
1) Headache, more right side than left – a familiar headache – thudding, but tingling as well, > pressing on it.
2) Tingling right foot.
3) Pain extends down right side of face, from head to neck.
4) Right hand colder than left.
5) Head, throbbing and twitching, right side. Right eye shifting in and out of focus. Hot around right eye, a little bit also on the left.
6) Right nostril feels heavy and blocked, wants to press on it. Like a whooshing sound down right nostril.
7) Feels the need to sleep.
8) Feels head leaning/going towards the right side, as if naturally.
(See prover no. 1 - headaches, page 33.)

> *To continue b.d. with the remedy for five days. Then to take an extra one if she finds herself wanting to cut her feet.*

17.01.07 *Phonecall.* Having strong headaches, in facial sinuses. Head leaning to the right in a fixed position. Painful, hence the phonecall. Tingling down arms and in feet, mostly right side. Slept very deeply after the first dose (05.01.07), otherwise sleep did not improve until last night. She slept right through, not waking at 4 a.m. She did take an extra tablet once re her feet. It was not immediately effective, but overall this urge has reduced sub-stantially again, from tds to once every few days.

17 01.07 *I advised one tablet (Pl.w 30) when the headache was severe.*

18.01.07 *Report.* Headache and leaning to one side, clear im-provement.

02.02.07 On the whole more positive. Pressing on right side si-nuses >. Also headaches in isolated patches > pressure.

Slept really well – not waking in middle of the night as much. Still having problems getting to sleep. Some nights no nightmares – progress; also a happy dream – very unusual.

More tired than before in the day. I feel I'm walking under wa-ter, everything is an effort. Memory loss. Fatigue. Clumsy.

I realised I was depending on alcohol to deal with stress. Not doing that now.

Feet cutting has not stopped but has been decreasing.

"When my partner started picking on me I held my own. Since the remedy I am not saying things just to make him happy.

I want an equal relationship."

02.03.07 Difficulties at work : Held my own. Surprised that I was able to hold eye contact. Proud of myself.

"For the first time - honest speaking with my grandparents about my Mum. They didn't make any comments about my weight, or judging what I do. I felt more relaxed. Also with my father, able to say what I want to do.

I feel lighter. I have broken free of my shackles. Before was settling for doing donkey work, couldn't complain.

Pl.w calms me down. Good at times of stress, like auditions. It helps a bit when I can't sleep; dreams are more vivid when I take it. Feet cutting still reducing.

Now, when I smile I smile completely. Now I have some mental space – like a tidy up, a spring clean in my head. Usually I see it as a messy place; now I can see the floor!

Pains in my body are moving down. Was head and neck, now right ovary and legs.

18.04.07 Rx. helped when I met up with my mother, but that lightness was shortlived.

06.06.07 *Pl.w had served its purpose. Staphisagria, Colocynth, Carcinosin and Aurum muriaticum natronatum followed.*

A concluding dream (of water) during this time: There were blocks of ice on wind streams above a calm moonlit sea – I was riding one of these blocks across the sea. Peaceful. Natural. Flowing. Pleasant. Someone in front of me started to slip. I helped her stand up. They were worried; I reassured her and helped her back.

This patient was doing well in some respects before I gave her Pl.w. As I see it, the particular impact of the remedy was in these areas of her life: feeling on an equal footing with her partner, able to sing, especially around him; self-harming, self-doubt, poor body image; beginning to see that her traumatic experiences could be faced and healed; ability to be seen by others, without a mask.

CASE 11

Female 20 years old D.O.B. 15.08.85

Pregnant; third month.

I use italics here to bring out the main features of her case (and the remedy).

Background: Energy and vitality : As a child, at least from her eighth year onwards and through her teens, she was mostly lacking in motivation. She would find it difficult to get up. There were headaches and stomach aches, especially on school days.

Being out in the world : She would be reluctant even to go to the corner shop on a simple shopping errand, as if not wanting to be seen in the world at large.

A central issue : As a teenager, as well as in the previous few years, she was much occupied with her appearance, clothes and make-up, and 'looking good', along with a underlying and deep-seated belief that she was not good-looking. She found good form for a while at a karate class; but in gradings and other such competitive tests, she would be very upset if she did not come out with the highest marks. She had some benefit from *Syphilinum*, (getting to sleep improved,) and *Aurum.* This helped her get through a dance exam. There is alcoholism and violence in the family history.

Alcohol use : She went through a time of frequent drinking in pubs and clubs. *Relationships* : From her early teens onwards, there has been a succession of boyfriends. Some have lasted for a few years, but on the whole, relationships with men have not been an easy part of her life.

She became pregnant very early on in her current relationship.

It was her mother who told me that she was pregnant and experiencing morning sickness. Knowing her history, I advised her to take *Plastic wrap 30 daily a.m.* and extras as required, if nauseous. She began this on 25.12.05.

12.01.06 She came to see me.

"Before the remedy I had some times of *dizziness:* it was

as if I would black out. I was walking around the supermarket and I felt if I didn't sit down I would faint. My head was reeling as if I had had too much to drink. Another time I felt dizzy in a similar way and went to sit on the toilet; it felt as if I would fall off the seat and I nearly did! Since taking the remedy this has not happened again."

Extra doses of the remedy helped at times of *feeling flustered,* or really tired or feeling a bit *nauseous.* (She was by now already past her first trimester, during which time the morning sickness had been more severe.)

Energy and waking in the mornings : "I'm waking now at 8.30 a.m. without an alarm. This is very unusual. Before it would be around 10 a.m., and even then I didn't feel like getting up. I used to feel groggy waking up; now I feel a lot fresher. I used to wake up and want to go back to sleep; now I am more wanting to wake up. Before I wouldn't feel tired till very late at night; now I get tired at 9 to 10 p.m. and want to go to bed. As long as I can remember I have had difficulty with sleeping. From what I've been told, from when I was two years old I found it difficult to get to sleep. Certainly since I was nine or ten years old I have never woken wanting to get up, till now."

Heartburn : Before the remedy, heartburn; in her upper chest, almost in her throat; heat and discomfort, < lying down, > sitting up. Scared to burp in case she might be sick. This cleared completely with the remedy, but had returned in the last few days, as did the nauseous feeling on waking. (She had run out of tablets three days before this session.)

Appetite and thirst : "Before, I was struggling with eating much; I didn't get hungry. I was only eating because I knew I had to, and the feeling of sickness wasn't helping. I can eat a bit more now. I have a definite sense of appetite again and know when I should eat. I am a little more thirsty." + Fizzy water and ginger ale type drinks.

Alcohol : She had already not been drinking much since the beginning of the pregnancy and for some time before that. "Maybe I have not wanted alcohol since the remedy. I only had one glass on New Year's Eve."

Relationships :

1) with her boyfriend: "Before, and especially since the pregnancy, I was reacting badly to him. The way he would sit on

the sofa in my Mum's house and go and fetch himself a glass of water without even asking; I thought he was being really rude behaving like that. I'd never do something like that in someone else's house! Since the remedy I am not bothered by this any more. All those things that would frustrate me, don't any more. I feel I'm back to that sense of being a new couple again."

2) with her family: "Since the remedy I have wanted to be around the family more, with my sister and her baby girl."

3) out and about in public places: "I am now finding all that less scary. For example, if I'm out, and someone that I don't know stops and says something to me, I am not so overwhelmed with it all. One time I felt faint in the supermarket. I took a tablet and began to feel better. I was sitting waiting for the others by the tills and a man who had finished his shift sat down next to me. He assumed I worked there too and started chatting to me. I was able to go along with his friendly chat; before I would have been too shy, not knowing how to respond. I would have thought that if I responded I would look and feel silly."

Supermarkets : Two of the previous occasions when she felt faint were in supermarkets. "I had to sit down or get away. I really wanted to go outside for fresh air, to get away from the atmosphere. I wanted to be left alone by everybody. I had to get myself a drink, I felt really hot. It was as if someone had come and taken away all your energy, sucked it out of you. My vision started to go fuzzy from the edges."

Skin : With the pregnancy she began to have spots on her face, big and aggressive. She had not had these teenage type spots before. Since the remedy they have calmed down.

12.01.06 *Rx: Plastic wrap 30 as required*, depending on her symptoms - nausea, heartburn, vertigo.

13.02.06 *Report: Nausea* >>. *Heartburn* : mostly goes by itself; twice when bad, Rx amel. *Skin* : Still spots, on left side of face. *Appetite* : Eating better still. *Alcohol* : not wanted any.

Relationships:

1) with the father of her child: "I have made a conscious decision not to be around him. He gets destructive around me. Before I would have got into arguments. Now I have more confidence to say I don't want to be around this."

2) with family: "I have been wanting to spend more time with people who are important to me and I am important to them,

for instance my family. I am finding it easier to get on with my sister. I am more tolerant of my Dad saying horrible things and he doesn't seem to be doing it so often."

3) out and about: "I have been noticing the public place thing. I am OK in other shops; it's just bad in places like clothes shops *(the volatile effect of plastics in synthetic clothes?)*, some buses, and shoe shops. I was in a shoe shop and had to go and sit down outside. Fuzzy eyes and light-headed again. It's to do with heat and claustrophobia – lots of people around. I needed the fresh air."

Waking up : "If I took the remedy in the morning previous to a day when I had to get up early for something, I would wake between 8.30 and 9.00 a.m. and felt able to get up; but if I took it in the evening when I didn't particularly want or need to get up early, I would wake feeling tired and wanting to go back to sleep."

Dreams : Of people I haven't seen since schooldays; people I haven't thought about for ages. *(School was difficult for her: peer pressures and influences.)*

How does life look now? "I feel more positive about the future. Maybe I'll go to college one day; something in the care way – midwifery or health visitor."

13.02.06 *Continue to use Rx as required.*

13.03.06. *Next appointment*

Nausea : Sick and sweaty on just one kind of bus. *(These new buses have a strong synthetic new fabric smell.)*

Supermarkets : "I take the remedy before I go in and I'm fine."

Heartburn : Bad again the last two days; Rx not tried yet, but will.

Carpal tunnel : New symptom since 2/52. Swollen, puffy, painful hands; base of fingers and the back of the hands. Right hand is worse – "I use it more. I can't make a fist." The pain is < clenching.

Headaches : The last two days. Little headaches that last for fifteen minutes. Middle of forehead and across eyebrows, < right side, > pressure, stroking the pain away.

Temperature and appetite : Since the pregnancy – not getting cold.

More hungry and eating bigger portions than before. "I'm happy now about the amount I'm eating." Wanting a more varied diet than before, + olives and + fish, − foods in sauces with meat in them, e.g. spagetti bolognaise or curries. Especially at the beginning of the pregnancy she would feel sick at the thought of them. Thirst? I feel thirsty more often. + Rooibosch tea.

Waking moods and energy : I'm waking early, 5.30 a.m., before daylight and I feel fine when I wake up. Moods generally OK.

Re father of the child : "He has disappeared. I'm fed up with him disappearing, thinking he can come and go when he pleases, but I know that because of his painful medical condition he has always had to think of himself first."

Re prospect of moving in with her sister : Feeling positive about it. "I like the idea of living with her."

13.03.06 *Rx: Plastic wrap 30, 3 doses in 24 hours, and then as required in case of heartburn or carpal tunnel symptoms.*

10.04 06 *Next appointment*

Remedy only needed recently once or twice a week and amel. each time. *Carpal tunnel* : before it was painful mornings on waking and evenings; now it comes on perhaps twice a week and only mildly.

Nights: Still waking 5.30 a.m., sometimes can get back to sleep. Sick in the night, the last two. Not much appetite in the last couple of days.

Dream : of having the baby in five seconds, at my father's house, and it was born the size of a year old baby.

Out and about: Now can get around a supermarket or have a short bus journey without having the remedy.

Relationship with father of the child : "Communication is better with him, although I haven't seen him, and don't want to yet. Before, when relationships have not been working, I would stay pissed off and shut down on it. I'm not doing that this time. Before, by not getting things out into the open and dealing with it, I was not letting myself get over it. Now I feel better about him, so instead of blocking him, I'm leaving it open to him to do what he will."

Gap of seven months.

03.07.06 Birth of baby girl.

30.11.06 *Next appointment* : Rx used quite a lot when she was first born; re heartburn and on the buses, then not needed at all.

Nausea/sickness: (Return of old childhood symptom.) Vomiting when on long car journeys, since the birth.

Appetite : Good, enjoying food.

Alcohol : Not had any for two months, then felt drunk after one glass of wine. Then in the night drank some squash and felt a bit dizzy again – like the heady thing of being drunk.

Multi-tasking and need to clean up : "I would get up to feed my daughter, then have her in the sling while I was washing up and then washing clothes. I can let things get to a certain point then I have to really clean up – not just tidy, but clean as well." *(Before she had not been a cleaning or tidiness person.)*

Periods : Recently restarted, possibly less painful since the birth.

Moods : "Since the birth of my daughter I have been a lot happier. Before at this time of year (Autumn) I would have got depressed."

Relationships with others : "I have dealt with things that were bothering me. I used to think 'Nobody likes me.' I don't think that way now. I am a lot less bothered what people think of me. Before, around my Dad I was so concerned about what he thought of me."

Going out : "Before, I would be happy to stay indoors and not go anywhere, ever; now I feel good going out at least once a day, if only to the shops. I don't like it if I haven't gone out in the day. I have more confidence in situations like asking people for directions. I was chatting to an old man in the bus; before I would have backed away from it. I took part in a group workshop. I was not expecting to hear it when others said how much they enjoyed working with me."

With the child's father: (This aspect of her relationships remains unresolved.) "It stays the same, and I feel uncomfortable about seeing him."

30.11.06 *Remedy suggestion: Plastic wrap 30 to take around the times she meets with him, and find out if it proves to be supportive.*

2008 review. She split up with the child's father and started another relationship.
In her subsequent pregnancy – successful use of Pl.w for morning sickness.
She is now married, in a much happier relationship, and is investigating courses in midwifery.

CASE 12

Female   D.O.B 16.04.89

This case spanning eight years recounts my first experience of prescribing Pl.w for a teenage girl.

Birth was very frightening for her mother; impersonal and unfriendly.

Aged 9
        First treated her when she was nine. At this time her mother was away each week for work, spending time with the family only at weekends. (She has a sister who is four years younger.) Her father brought her to see me (about hearing problems), and along with au pairs or nannies he takes care of the two girls during the week. The set-up was already established when my client was much younger, and continued, in essence well into her teens.
        Significant aetiology, as I understand it: her relationship with her mother.
        Fathers description: cerebral child, cut off with it, tends to live in a world of her own. Sensitive especially to criticism, or being told what to do. Shouting fights. Tears. "She won't do anything her mother tells her to do."
        Her response after *Thuja*, "I'm all broken up into pieces and there's no-one to pick me up. This is gong to last forever and I'm going to be embarrassed all my life." No trust.

137

Aged 11

She returned concerned about a wart below her left knee.

Recurring dream: *(theme of water)* "At a place like Centre Parks. I just sneak out onto the balcony to a place where it is sunny. Then to a swimming pool (it is dark now) and in the darkness, a man with a cap and uniform is sweeping a bit of water away. I get onto a slide, go down a bit and stop, and that's where my dream ends. In my dreams I'm happy to go down the slide, but in real life I don't like things like roller coasters, giant slides or heights, I don't like the feeling of falling."

After *Thuja 1M* her dreams of falling stopped but her dreams of water continued along with other themes; these included "lots of dreams of girls and women that I knew."

Another of her dreams of water: enormous swimming pools. "There is an area at the top that is smaller and less deep, and then there is a more deep water in the bigger pool. I don't go into the deep pool. There the water hurts you if you go under it. I am in an area that doesn't hurt you, and I only go in up to my legs. The men in the dream are quite evil and want to hurt you. They were mostly quite old. If you stayed in the deep water too long it would hurt you like the radiation of TV."

Father's report to me at this time: She has difficulties relating to school friends. She talks and wants them to listen, but is not prepared to listen much. This makes them annoyed with her. She is worried about not having friends, and is withdrawing into herself. She is picked on and bullied with all of this. When she is not being bullied so much, she feels excluded by the others.

Her confidence improved with *Calcarea carbonica 1M*. She was still quiet and not confident at school for fear of being bullied, but was getting on better with her friends.

Nightmare: "Trying to get away from someone and then outside it was sunny and nice. Then I saw a woman who had a mask(?) on and she was tugging on it slowly to pull it off." *(Compare Case 10 re masks, especially page 127.)*

Gap of two years.

Aged 14 (no periods as yet).

About school work, which dominates her life: "Now I am not

really choosing what I want to do, and I feel guilty if I have fun. Not much sense of enjoyment."

About friends: "I worry about friends and what they think of me. I'm never really sure if they really like me. Everything they say I analyse and put it in a bad way. My head does that. I feel left out when they play cards and I don't know how to play."

Dream: "Of being two years older and my sister has weird hair, blonde and stuck up."
I feel anxious and embarrassed about everything.
Calcarea carbonica 1M again.

Less bothered about school work, managing it better, not worrying now about school friends. "They sometimes shut me out but I know they don't mean to. It doesn't matter what they think of me. I've just got to get on with it.

I'm getting upset about feeling fat. I snack through the day and feel guilty and bad about doing it. I feel ashamed and worried about my body. If I have a problem and my mother is a bit harsh, I think, 'It doesn't matter, it will go away'. My father will give me support."

After *Pulsatilla 200* and then *Medorrhinum americanum 200,* father's report: She is a lot happier. She has put behind her the issues of food and growing larger, she is not snacking so much and eating healthier food. Not so much angst about things, or teenage moodiness.

Aged 15. Periods have now started.

Can now focus on things at school and works really hard, but not looking for an academic future. "I want to do girly things, be a housewife and have children. With all the school work I feel my enthusiastic side has been buried.

I can get annoyed with my child-minder. I don't like her looking after me. It can be that there is no one to talk to in my house and my friends don't seem to understand.

Annoyed/frustrated if cannot find nice clothes in shops. Bothered about my appearance and wanting to look slender."

I considered Pl.w. for her. (The proving had begun three months before this.) I didn't give it yet.

Aged 16

Miserable. Lot of pressure from school and family. Homework seems so hard. "Recently I can wake feeling panicky, once or twice a week. I want to run away. Then in five minutes it's OK. I'm fine once I get to school and see my friends. With the panic I feel miserable, angry and desperate. It doesn't happen if I'm woken by the alarm."

Main concerns: "Social life is hard, frustrating. I don't have the friends I want to have; those with similar interests and ideas; and I feel I should have friends outside of school and a boyfriend. I seem to be busy all the time but still not getting enough done. What would I like to be doing more of? Dancing to music videos, more social occasions with friends, parties, getting drunk, swimming, gym."

Again some improvement after *Calcarea carbonica 30*. Not nervous but in other ways worse.

Feel self-conscious, chubby trying on clothes.

"My mother always pressurises me to do everything, and fast. She piles on everything for me to do. If I get fed up and complain about things she says, "Stop being so silly". I have to do everything my parents tell me. I spend so much time making others happy. It never feels like I'm working for myself.

Carcinosin 30, weekly for six weeks, helped: "I've been sleeping better and it's easier to get to sleep. I feel more happy and spend less time worrying. The pressure is less intense so I feel more relaxed. Before I was changing because others wanted me to change – now they don't mind me changing."

Then paradoxically : "I'm feeling less and less secure. It's getting harder and harder at college and I'm not as relaxed generally as I used to be. It's difficult socially and I feel like my college work is getting pushed to one side. I feel restless when I sit down to do work. I'm getting less sleep in general; it's as if I have lost my balance."

I ask about the difficulties of her social life.

"Sometimes it feels like everyone else has a boyfriend. I have real trouble interacting with boys. Maybe I'm just attention seeking. With guys I might be around them in ways that feel really exciting and fun, then it just stops. With one girl in my class all I'm envious of is the things she can do well socially.

When she's talking all the guys are naturally attracted to her. God made her that way – she has a boyfriend, and lots of others falling in love with her.

Generally I have moods, I get really excited, then sad, restless and hopeless. At first it's like running on a treadmill, than it's as if I get off and feel weird: everything stops. In myself I feel empty. I keep on rushing to do things, hoping it will be all right. I feel shut off from other people a bit. I think the real me isn't very nice. I try to get peoples' attention, demanding of it: I can be brash in what I say, being quite loud. I'm talkative and don't leave gaps. I sometimes act and feel like a child. My cousin says that my Mum babies me, a lot later than normal; my mother wasn't around when I was little so I'm emotionally under-developed.

Feeling abandoned is an issue for me; e.g. if people go off line (on MSN) or I have made friends with guys and then they don't want to be friends with me. I'm not so comfortable on my own as I was. I attract bad friendships with guys. With one guy I clicked, we were like brother and sister, then he wasn't interested, he had a girlfriend.

I've been having weird dreams. In one of them my father died. I was coming home from college, walking home. A few people were standing outside the house with the door open. One of them (a woman) said he had died. Then I was screaming and the woman said, "Please don't be upset, you are making me upset". I saw him dead on the floor, he looked so peaceful.

My sleep is restless. When I wake it feels like I haven't been asleep for a long time.

When I go out with friends I put on clothes that suit me. I look pretty and I feel relaxed, but I feel out of place because I can't be friends with Chavs. If I dressed like them, and played the same music as them, it would make it easier for me, but I like what I wear and the music I like. It's harder to make friends because I wouldn't fit in easily. I would have to fake it and would feel more self-conscious in those clothes. I'd be like an imposter if I wear their fashion clothes.

I feel nervous inside my gut. It can be when I wake in the morning and I'm dreading the day ahead. It's like how I feel in exams. I dread things, I haven't done this piece or that piece of work. About half the time I feel uneasy like this when I wake up, but not at weekends.

I wish I could be like the girl with loads of friends and get attention without being overly dramatic. I feel I have to be dramatic or no one will give me attention."

02.02.06 *Remedy given in session: Plastic wrap 30*
Initial response: "My head feels clearer."
Then two more doses night and morning, and to repeat if nervous tummy returns after an improvement.

24.02.06 *She has a shining quality, and presents herself with a new ease.* She recalls feeling calmer for a day or two. Not the nervous feeling in her tummy.

She had taken the remedy 6th, 11th and 12th February; and felt better for a couple of days each time.

She has had a stabbing pain in her heart area, two or three seconds each time. It stopped her in her tracks. R.O.S. similar to previous pains which she had had elsewhere as well as around her heart. *Place of stored grief?*

She felt calmer when on a family holiday, less attention seeking, but she is usually better in this respect when not at college. But even at college things were different, especially when she was feeling calmer. "I felt I appeared more together. I was holding something back in an interesting way. I was worrying less about what people thought.

Since the remedy I've been happier – it didn't matter what I was wearing. A week ago for a party my friend dressed me up how they dressed up. I wore skinny jeans for the first time in my life, and nice little shoes. They put eye make-up on me. It was nice to look nice and feel prettier. Lots of girls have to dress up smutty to make boys notice them – it's nice not to have to think like that.

Before in the class I would be bothered about trying to get this guy's attention, now I'm not bothered.

It's an adjustment, switching away from the little child mode. It will take a long time to do this. If I realise I have the same emotions as everyone else it is better than feeling different."

Dream: "I was pregnant. I had just found out. I was so freaked out that I was pregnant and didn't want a baby. So scared. A year ago I had a dream of being pregnant and walking around with a massive belly, happy and sunny. A fantasy state at that time.

I slept better for a while, but I have felt more tired in the day. This goes with being less attention seeking.

It's been good to go out and do things while I'm not necessarily so involved with my friends: things they don't know I do. I went jogging last night, first time in ages; at first I felt puffed but then it felt really good. Running relatively fast felt really fun. Thrashing it out (with loud music on headphones) makes me feel calmer when I finished.

I want to have more tact, to be less childish and less showy-offy, but not one of those people who are slightly boring.

I keep seeing magpies around but mostly only one. That's not nice, they are supposed to come in pairs."
Then we saw two in the garden outside the clinic window!
I asked her to remind me of the rhyme associated with magpies:

"One for sorrow, two for joy
Three for a girl, four for a boy,
Five for silver, six for gold,
Seven for a secret, never to be told."

Father's report : She is *much* happier around the house and more positive. She even offered to come dancing with me at the salsa class!
24.02.06 *Rx: Pl.w. 30 One a week for four weeks.*

Aged 17
I did not see her for ten months. She had felt better for several months, but not so good now.
20.12.06 "I am at a new college, in another town. It's as if I have gone back years. I have reverted back to wanting my classmates' attention. I feel so unconfident and unattractive there. I used to feel more confident. I feel more confident in my home city, and with old friends. Boyfriends? I don't feel pretty at all or that I have a nice personality.

I liked Christmas with my family. I don't have to make an effort. They won't let me get too much into myself - thinking a lot. It's nice to have honest people, people who care – they so much want the best for you. They overlook your faults. I don't have to worry about being too boring or too interesting: I'm just one person. I miss the family connections when I'm not with them.

It got to the point when I was thinking everything was going to be all right, then I went to this new college. I've not been happy for ages. I feel totally at odds with myself. I used to be worried after meeting new friends that I wouldn't see them again; now I am not interested in making new friends at college. I get bored. The people are boring and dull, especially the girls. No social graces. People out in that place act on a certain level. I get irritated: for example with girls that have horrible hair and don't take care of it. I am more myself with my old friends.

I feel less confident out around the place and around other people: what if others think that me and my group of friend are boring? I don't mind if they think we are bitchy or self-centred. They have pretty faces, nice hair and clothes, but nothing behind it.

It bothers me if some college work goes badly – there's no one to talk to about it. My mother *(living with the family through the week now)* is not motherly; she's more like a friend who gets mad at you over something.

What stops you being the real you? I don't think I can ever be that with anyone else apart from my real family. My biggest fear is that I'm boring. With my family, they don't care about little details, they wholly accept me. With friends, I do feel quite accepted and valued; with other people, I don't feel accepted. They decide if I'm good enough for them. I don't accept others. I decide whether they are good enough for me.

I see some people, like at a party. How can I not get happiness etc? They can, and they are so dull.

People mistake what I say or do for confidence; but that's not who I really am.

I take things so personally: about weight, appearance and clothes issues. I am really paranoid about weight and appearance when it is talked about in general. I never thought I was pretty. I think others don't think I'm pretty.

After I first had that remedy *(Plastic wrap)*, I filled in more *(sic)* in myself, I was a better version of myself: like when you get a really nice hair cut or nice new clothes. I fit more into

myself. Now, I feel like I'm outside and viewing myself from outside, like through a camera."
20.12.06 *Rx: Pl.w 1M, split dose.*

07.02.07 I spoke to her father, who told me how things had been
in the intervening six weeks: "Definitely better. Not long after
the remedy she had a 'great fight' with her mother. This clarified
things and now they are getting on well. College work is going
OK; she is cheerful and looks healthy and happy."

CASE 13
In this case Plastic Wrap is the first and main remedy.

Female. 40 years old. D.O.B. 03.07.65
Screen-play writer since 16 years old. Lives with partner and
their two young children, aged four and two.

Sick regularly. Stomach gets really bloated. Swollen and
painful - hypochondria - but only 6-8 p.m. onset; > if lies down
flat with knees up. Rubbing relieves it; passing wind relieves it.
More likely to come on or << when hasn't eaten anything. Cramping pain and round to back. Has had these symptoms since mid-
20's.
Also bowel thing for many years — three times since age
22 and a small version recently (from tea). Like a panic attack
and everything comes out: diarrhoea and vomiting, shaking, cold
and shivering; otherwise tends to constipation, since early twenties.
History of leaky gut before children were born, also cold
and flu symptoms. History of Candida - spots on foot, and it can
get into mouth. Has done Candida diet and OK if off all sugars
and alcohol to minimum.
When gets run down, not sleeping through night re children. It's all too much: needing to hibernate. Two young boys.
Cleaning house and writing career. Energy can't sustain it, as if no
choice. Wiped out evenings and weekends.
I want to do exercise, but it wipes me out. Yoga, self nurturing, to give myself the time.
Periods : PMT badly aged 17-18 for two years. At that

time, I remember feeling unworthy, not good enough; I hated my physicality, body bloated with water, breasts enormous, painful – (more recently, since birth of second child, no PMT and not much pain). It was an appearance issue in my eyes. I was supposed to be the beautiful one, the actress; my sister the intelligent one. Always felt ordinary, plain and stupid and not the clever one. Pushed myself to get A's to prove myself. Feelings of unworthiness.

Childhood : Mother left father when I was eight, to father's best friend. The most painful thing was that we weren't allowed to cry in any way - my emotions not important, expression not important.

Family context : F didn't accept me. M having affairs when I was three. M is 70 and fit - has had thyroidectomy. F died of cancer six years ago - he was 60. An alcoholic. M's M – nothing was ever said or expressed. No connection with my M. My M was sent to boarding school at five. She hated her nanny.

Childhood illnesses. Antibiotics for earache. Tonsillitis a few times. Glands up and down. Had vaccines. No childhood illnesses (like chicken-pox or whooping cough). Had fevers.
(*I thought of Carcinosin.*)

How do you feel just now? Uneasy. Shoulder tension. Compression below rib cage.

Being perfect Mum doing everything and anything – I try to make up for being unworthy. It's exhausting – I want to run away – not to be with the kids. Overwhelmed, almost panicky - impatient - afraid will hurt them. Physically I shake and get palpitations. Sleep is often bad: lack of sleep, broken sleep - since four and a half years.

Dreams: nothing repeating. In the past, of me, waitressing. Anxiety dreams around this - food not coming in time. As actress, forgetting my lines on stage. Re not having belief in myself to carry it through. Not being fast enough, not good enough. To prove I can handle it. Of not being attractive enough. Couldn't socialise or do other bits that needed to do.

I have a sister - she is the concert pianist; I was the actress. As an actress I could express my feelings of anger etc. freely. I was angry for a really long time.

Stepfather - an ogre. He tried to kill us sometimes. Violent and verbally abusive. Used to dye my hair black to get attention from other men. F - when went to see him, I felt so ugly, fat and stupid. Appearance a big thing. Big thing about me in relation to men - I was late having my first relationship. It was with an older man. I was his princess. Never trusted men.

I have just written a Cinderella script for a film. *By now my thoughts of Pl.w as a Rx were confirmed! See The Cinderella Connection Page 180.*

How are you in the house? Things have to be clean - otherwise frustrated, annoyed, unsatisfied. Always up to me to do it all. In most areas I find it difficult to ask people to do things. Gets it clean - all those hours - then bothered a few days later. When they are clean and tidy I can breathe and think. Comfortable in those circumstances.

With alcohol? Alcohol — I get an instant headache, and a hangover two hours later.
I don't drink much water. I drink red bush tea - comforting.
How is your tummy just now? Its tense, gurgling - mild version of usual afternoon symptoms.
02.03.07 *Rx: Pl.w 200 given in session.*
Reaction: Stomach has stopped gurgling. It feels a bit soothed. Stomach area peaceful, quiet. Open now. Was protected.
Same Rx to take in case of her usual evening stomach symptoms.

08.03.06 *Phone report.* Five days of constant pain a.m. and night. Last two days not a problem in the night. *Pl.w 200* again 3rd March, 5th March, then no pains in the night.

20.03.06. *Second appointment.* Evening tummy things not happening at all now.

When I have to deal with other people or rather deal with myself with other people in unfamiliar environment, I become tense and self-conscious. Nervous re wanting it to be perfect, eloquent, impressive - to say right thing. Now I'm wanting to be real, very much more. Feels like I'm present. I'm listening. I'm not self-conscious.

Home life : Managed it > than have before. Even-keeled, stable - even when under lot of family pressures and didn't lose it. Not felt so overwhelmed by household things, but yesterday it felt hard to let go of doing it - people coming issue.

Menses : painful this time - more than recently. Familiar

sensations – and on time. Since last pregnancy has had no PMT.

No shakes, palpitations, panic.   Constipation - remains. Doesn't really clear. Dry skin. (Since the remedy.) Like sandpaper.

After first Rx - began to think about impact of early years and father's divorce; my brother and I went with our mother. Sister was left behind. All these kind of things. Emotionally I haven't gone there, because it's painful.

Day two of menses, wanting just to be with me, not needing to get away. I'm becoming integrated with the world. Asking for what I needed used to be difficult for me.
20.03.06 *Rx. use Pl.w. 200 as required.*

21.04.06
(She was treated on the phone by my locum in this instance.)

Two weeks of nausea - not eating - very tired with headache too. A bit better today. Nausea not better for eating. Wanting brown rice, simple food. Bloated, cramping, rumbling; > first thing in morning, < when gets up. Feels heavy, wants to hide away - withdraw. *Rx: Sepia 30. Tds 2/7.*

28.04.06 Stomach calm. Less tired. Less withdrawn.

A gap of seven months.

November '06. I have been fine since April. I realised that I got the stomach upsets every time I was in an environment where I was uncomfortable within myself.

Any more thoughts about the past? To do with myself: The place I was at when I was twenty. I go back to that place because I felt worthless. Didn't want to leave the house because of how I felt about myself. Not intelligent. Not attractive enough. Won't succeed in what I want to do. Like a dark time.

What makes things worse these days? When I'm very tired and unwell - can go into this place - can last for a minute or two. Sad when I go there. I feel different for having a better understanding of myself. Can step out of it with words and understanding.

Re relationships with men? More comfortable now. Don't feel stupid - can hold my own now. Before didn't speak for fear of being stupid - also with girl friends - but with girl friends not fitting in, didn't belong - with men - not good enough and attractive - stupid, therefore not loveable.

With the children? Constantness of being present with them - it's tough. Gets inspired by work and want to remain in it. Struggle to find balance is the issue - wanting to be with them to be perfect mother and always fall short - bad mother. Has had time on my own - peace was so nurturing. If not well and tired can be irritable and I get a surge of anger - when the elder one of the boys hurts his younger brother - he thumps him: triggers something of my childhood - injustice.

Writing second draft of Cinderella film script. My struggle is finding time to finish that.

CASE 14
A case with many dreams.

Female aged 42. D.O.B. 04.04.64

06.04.05 First appointment

M.E.

Headaches - Every location as if throughout. Feels hard holding head up, often as if falling to left. < Noisy places. Can be < too much bright sunlight. Light feels like an onslaught. Eyes ache with headache; >> cranial people holding head. Always sensitivity around head. Mum hit me/pulled my hair.
Generally on waking - grogginess, like a bad hangover.

Abdominal discomforts: flatulence, churning. Nauseous. Cramps. Unsettled bowels.

I am the third of six children. After I was born, my mother had post-natal depression. I remember my mother being unpredictable. Suicide attempts after sixth child. My mother says that my birth was 'very easy', but she will think things are OK when they are not. Breast fed for three months, not much milk. Don't think it was a joyful thing for her. My mother was good in practical taking care of things, not emotional things.
I have had two terminations. Miscarriage 2001.

Vaccinations - lots. Childhood and travel.
Tonsillectomy aged 8. Lots of tonsillitis.
Hungry for touch and holding.
Re M.E. - Angry and let down by my physical body, not what it's supposed to do.

What do you feel were the effects on you of your mother's violence? I was not sensitive to bodily needs; for a long time I had no idea how to rest: bit removed from body. Absent from pelvic area, sexually dysfunctional, disconnected, not dropped down into myself. Not relaxed. Turbulent inside. Brother sexually abused me once. I was seven, he was two years older. My early relationships were abusive. Mother would say horrible things to me or not talk to me for days on end. I was a burden: she didn't want me around.

Picking at skin around fingers, quite severe. Will do this at times of great distress.

Recent dreams:

1) Mother thought I was disgusting and smelly and pushed me away.

2) Doing a performance. M didn't come or to take me home.

3) Familiar flavour: having to escape from dangerous situation, unseen force, e.g. in bomb damaged city and have to get somewhere safe.

4) I have a penis that has been cut off. Several other people in this position. One handed to me that was supposed to be mine. Confused. Don't know why this has happened. Don't want to be identifying which is mine. Feels gruesome. Disempowerment?

5) Of helping children under ten to escape. Urgency/anxiety. Leading them through countryside. Looking for a route to take them to safety.

6) About my Mum with her in the house where I grew up. Seething with frustration at her. Pushing her and pinching her in the face to get a reaction. She wasn't responding at all. Full of frustration and rage. Familiar dream - and waking experience. It is impossible to have a meaningful connection with her. She lives in Canada - quite estranged.

These days it feels like I'm coming out of something. Letting go of some of expectations of family. Not locked in. Feel more fluidity about it. Determination to break away from shackles of unfulfilled longing. I'm in the conduit. Expression of what others are not feeling.   M.E. linked to this.

Can't sleep re not feeling safe - fear someone might hurt me in the night - hit me - sexual thing is in there. Can't switch off. *Sleep improved later on with Ferrum muriaticum. See below.*

Dream : Yew trees filling the garden - dense canopy. Feels magical under them. Liked it that something I had planted had grown and created something quite magical.

06.04.05 *Rx: Buddleia 30 twice a week 4/52 and Nux vomica 12 daily 4/52.*

Dream : By the sea in small cottage. Out of window see small family group playing in high water. I go out to see if it is safe. Later tide is out and I see that it's safe to jump in the water. For now I've missed my chance and will have to see if it's safe next time tide goes out. Then by a river and a man is carrying a boy across water, dark and deep water. It's a dream of taking the plunge but not quite yet. Out into the world.

Hatred of mother when father left. I was seven. Very aware of lack of fathering. He wasn't around to protect me from hurt of M and he was wanting someone to be the most special young woman. Angry with father and stepmum.

Dream : Mum evicting me from family house, me needing to be supported after that and sister ignoring me.

Dream : M and one of brothers walking along arm in arm and telling her how angry I am. She didn't love me enough and abandoned me. I punch her stomach. Others in family angry too. Anger is why I've been sidelined. She didn't answer me back - just listened.

Doubt about being functioning human being and out in the world. Stuck in my restrictions, when is this thing going to properly change? - feelings of isolation. Left behind - left out in the cold.

22.09.05 *Rx: Ferrum muriaticum 30 daily 2/52.*

Effects of Ferr. mur. : Positive. Sleeping better. *(First time in her treatment that sleep improved.)*

Dream after Ferr. mur. : Of seeing a newt in compost in kitchen - tried getting it out - it became bigger, eg lizard/komodo dragon, must take it to wild/zoo. In plastic bag - see it's too squashed - very worried for its survival - concerned about specialness of it.

Back really sore as it often is. Sacrum at the root, sore and fragile. Need to strengthen abdominal muscles - movement very difficult - wary of movement. Very little strength in back. Injury inflicted by Mum - upper lumbar area damaged.
30.01.06 *Rx: Conium IM*

After *Conium*, good experience in meditation - sublime - fantastic. Of feeling really integrated top and bottom of body - through the middle of me.

Dream : A fountain of love coming up through my body. Soft and abundant feeling.

Dream : The anxious type. Of travelling, missing times, connections, not ready, not going to make it. In midst of travelling - train or bus - can't speak language, can't get information, don't know what the time is, so have missed connection. Rushing to next stage and think I've missed it. Don't find outcome of it.

Connection: re Dad - his job was to travel - passenger jet travel - lot of anxiety around this. When little, a lot of coming and going, insecurity and broken attachment. Gets stressed, leading to departure and making arrangements. Lead up is worst. OK when travelling.

Where in your body do you feel this anxiety?

Stomach. Tension in stomach. Not allowing ease of digestion through knot where I feel the anxiety and stress, also overwhelm feeling; also shoulders achy.
04.03.06 *Rxs: Pl.w 30. 11.03.06, Pl.w 200. 18.03.06, Pl.w IM.*

30.03.06 *Report* : First two doses (30 + 200) - breaking down in tears two days later, out of the blue - brought up anxiety that had been in dreams before. Lot of feeling insecure/anxious: socially inadequate, overwhelmed with complexities of life and fearful of future. World felt dangerous and frightening as well as confusing: life wouldn't be tenable. Global warming/wars. My life wouldn't be tenable as well as the world's existence.

L. side head - phlegmy - thick, mornings, for ten days to two weeks – like a cold.

Dream, night of Pl.w 30 : Church with priest and small group of family near altar. Brother was given a pill. He swallows it and falls down dead. Everyone impassive. I'm deeply shocked that he was there one minute and not the next and no one does anything.

Dream of looking after younger siblings, stressful; time pressure to make food.

And your long-term symptoms? Every day I wake with a head-ache; not so bad last few days re better sleep.

Dream : a few days after Pl.w 30 : with younger siblings in wild trying to find somewhere to stay. Sleeping on rocky ledges - afraid might be wild animals around. This changes to . . . Indonesia - drives car into temple - embarrassed. I go to apolo-gise to monks - one gives me a monkey (toy). Helping children to make duck noises so that they will know how to get food and be safe . . . re-entering temple with a man, my partner - telling him how much I love him . . . to town to pilgrims' quarters . . . in a very dangerous place - in a nuclear reactor given a tour. ? with brother - very scared.

Dream : at a small frozen lake, with friends. Climb up tower - as I walk up it dislodges and about to topple across the lake - to hit the other shore. I jump - breaking the ice into deep clear water - unharmed. Someone says how brave I am. My feeling: "Well it's turned out all right." More oceanic now, not a shallow pool.

Dream : anxious re travel and getting food - not enough money, not getting food I need etc.

Dream - two days after Pl.w 200 : Horse dream. Arrive in middle of night in a city. Raining. Walking the streets - need to find somewhere to stay. Come to a café. Think I should get a friend and come back. Then with a horse on the stairs - large, powerful and in distress. Chestnut bay. I'm trying to soothe it - hard. Also I'm anxious about my situation. Horse/person. Hold-ing it really close to me, talking to it. It feels as if it is a small child that has lost the horse. Have to hold it until it calms down. Really love this horse - tell it I love it - eventually it believes me and it relaxes. I know this horse has suffered a lot in the past. Then go with companion to find a woman's house - long time to find bearings - so late we will have missed her. Companion has lost horse; he was supposed to be looking after it, also lost car keys. We have to go back to find them, knowing where to look.

Had felt good the day after the 200. Felt quite clear, with steady energy. Quite connected - to other people - more peace-

153

ful, integrated. Then horse dream - next day my back was very sore. Gardening set it off. Next day, stroppy/short-tempered - burst into tears and felt better. At first too much to handle, then releasing. Lot of grief came to the surface - possibly the whole well. Feeling full of grief. There has always been grief, always will be totally overwhelming. Some current, some not.

Dream two days after Pl.w 1M : of being in a church - a boy aged 13/14. (He is like my ex.) Taking him there for his baptism. I'm responsible for him. Our pew fills with other people (? siblings) and priest is late.

Dream, connected with the previous one : with two younger brothers, twins aged seven, in a bathroom. One of them is in the water - lying on his back underwater and looks drowned. I pick him out of water - his body is still and I carry him to the next room. I want to throw him to the ground to bring him back to life. I pump his chest and he comes back - but I'm not sure he wants to be alive.

Dream : of meeting my ex in the street. (Not seen him for four years. Since then he has had a child.) Very happy to see him. Child (boy, six months) with him. I'm carrying his son - asking him how he's getting on with parenthood. Walking down the street - very painful to have to give the baby back to him. Tears. (I actually saw him today.)

We grew up together. Together for seven years: exciting life together travelling, working abroad. Thought it would be for ever. At time of disclosure in family (about abuse) - so much distress and trauma - didn't know what I was doing – I had an affair. I was frustrated that he (my ex) wouldn't go 'beneath the surface'. I was quite cruel - regret how I treated him - over years - harboured secret desire that our lives could be entwined.

Abdomen: feeling > till about a week ago. More stable. Bowels functioning >. Less flatulence. Better movements, not so bloated, uncomfortable. Last week haywire again. Churning/nauseous; feeling hungry and nauseous all the time, crampy. Now just past ovulation. Slight vaginal infection - last ten days, slight fishy odour - unusual - not for ages.

30.03.06 *Rx: Pl.w 1 M in session. Response* : Tummy - gas comes up and softer in there – but still edgy.

A gap of eight months.

06.12.06 Looking back at these months - connections re Plastic wrap: feeling of not having skin on my body - too sensitive. Overloaded sensorily. Whole system can't cope. With remedy: brighter in myself, a bit. Physically not much change. Now the feeling of being too sensitive is more distant, i.e. I feel more resilient. Old symptoms around, but not so strong.

Dream : 30.03.06 - *the day of the last dose of Pl.w 1M. (She had kept a diary record since our previous session.)* Estranged brother in dream. *(The brother that had abused her.)* Feel awkward when he comes to house. Reluctantly let him in. I am a lodger in a friend's house. It's a chaotic house in the country. Can't stand the chaos. Group of young teenagers upstairs. Musicians, ? men, arrive. Feel invaded; positive side is creativity out of chaos. Before dream: restless limbs, and shouting in sleep.

Dream : 02.04.06. With people I don't know very well in flat. Feeling scared and vulnerable. Anything could happen. Violence to me?

Dream : 03.04.06. In house with M and siblings. She is running a brothel upstairs. It's very dangerous here. Man comes to door at night. I shout to M to warn her that he has a weapon. Too late. He has a hatchet. Throws it. It goes right through another woman who is in front of my mother, and imbeds in mother's stomach. He then has a gun and is going to shoot me. Trying to phone. Phones don't work. I go to hide in loo - unsuccessful. Phone calls, 999 etc. Impending mortal danger. Inability to get help. M not being helpful in any way. TYPICAL. Then wound on body. L side abdomen. Second vulva, numb not sensitive. Uncomfortable, needs cleaning.

Looking back over the months since taking the remedy (Pl.w) I've not had so much of wounded dreams - myself or others. There has been a change in my typical dreams of driving and not being in control: I have had others with me and it's not so dangerous.

08.04.06 *Dream* : In big building. Department store. On hospital bed. Siblings around. Others in hospital beds. Slipping under with anaesthetic. Then woken by man. Forcing food into my mouth. Also shaking ankles violently. When come round surgery had not been performed on me - was to have been on my gut. They are on the run - dangerous. Huge mass of people trying to get out of building - it feels very unsafe.

14.04.06. *Dream* : Nairobi - car brakes down. Men start hassling me. Frightened so I hide - they pass by. Then - as a teenager at male friend's house. Strange kite-like creature (from Lord of Rings) comes down to get us with its claws. Manage to get away, but it's wounded. Friend's father returns - realise I've fallen in love with him. Very dangerous. Would cause problems for others and wife.

Dream : Mid-June. Car brakes not working. Going downhill backwards in the dark, but someone is with me.

Dream : recent, of going through countryside in daylight with air under feet - with someone, a man partner. Side by side, in control. Quite high up, could see over hedges - going fast.

Dream : most recent - I did rescue a drowning baby. Picked her out of water and to side of pool. I thought she was OK. Lifeguards had to ressuscitate her. Was she OK? Or not.

Dream of a daimon, a cat - freaked out - claws. Out shopping – cat has to go in basket; in the countryside – to fight/mating. Stressful to hold her and keep her safe. Fear car will hit her.

Dream : in car. Night. Captive. Man (my lover) has violent intentions. Fighting with him. Futile. Desperate. Then three people, dismembered.

Reflecting on these dreams - Underlying fear of being thwarted by people. Easily threatened. Also by sound, e.g. on buses - can't stand those noisy environments. Sensitivity to toxicity - smell/sounds. In the Autumn I didn't feel well - more M.E. type symptoms.

Now there are changes: things have opened up in my life. Cabaret performance to people - growing more. Loving it. Course on improvised comedy. Feels well. Connected. It doesn't take any energy. Playful. Silly. Slightly saucy but endearing. When doing it, it feels absolutely fine. Very connecting with other people. In a beam of light. That goes through me down into the ground.

Sleep generally not bad. Before one good night in fifty, now mostly good nights.

CASE 15

These are notes from phone consultations. I had sent the remedy to this friend to take. He was so often tired and stuck with his circumstances. Knowing him and the remedy I suggested that Plastic wrap might make a difference. He is a musician.

Male aged 64 D.O.B. 15.07.42 He is in a relationship.

10.01.06 *Rx: Plastic Wrap 200, 3 in 24 hours.*
12.01.06 *Phone report.* Lot more energy suddenly last night. Not tired after rehearsal, unusual.

Sleep: usual waking around 5 a.m., but not worrying as much as before. Immobility and procrastination has always been around fear, e.g. to get on with income tax; feels more ready to do that now. Surprise is that things went well - arrangements for the rehearsal had stuck - could remember them well. Not unusual - what was unusual was not being afraid of not knowing them.

23.01.06 Even although worried about money, sleeping through 5 a.m. now.

Greatest procrastinator ever. Lack of prioritising. Loss of sense of proportion e.g. as a diversionary tactic, fixing the light bulb rather than getting down to the tax return. Has to get act together for concerts in March. Lays there worrying about all of it. Since Rx moments of huge despair. Since the last two weeks – interacting with people more, despite what's going on.
23.01.06 *Rx: Repeat Pl.w 200*

01.02.06 Basically very good. Main thing is lot more energy. Eating better. Energy, in spite of doing things that before would have set me back a couple of days. Not so much despair. Sadnesses - realistically based but do not take over. Determination is better. When a teenager I would normally not do things for school till last minute, then do them half-assed; but this work has to be ready for a music tour. Felt more self-contained around other musicians - not that worried about it. Still felt usual paranoia, but didn't disable me out of proportion.

After I took the last tablet I managed to keep on working at something; before would have stopped. Waking at 5 a.m. Intensity of anxiety is less. Finding it easier to get on with things - before was paralysed.

School days were all like this. I live on fear. Failure at getting things done on time - so it would swamp me when I start to do something. Taking this remedy brings on this reminder of fear. Reminder of when younger I used to deliberately keep myself tired and separate from everyone.

Usually would fret about small administrative difficulties and now not. Energy > re moving out of a depressed state. I was playing the violin in a quartet - it really worked - like coming into a clearing in a beautiful place and reacting to it. Before, when driving, a lot of times I had to stop and take a rest - not this time since Rx. Panic less.

Gap of a year.

09.01.07 *After those first tablets the improvement lasted for three months.*
Now feeling stuck with things and low energy.
Rx: Pl.w 200, 3 in 24 hours.

18.01.07. *Report.* After first of three tablets. Woke 7 a.m. A lot going on. Money issues are a constant torture. Sleep again and woke 9.30 a.m. Day 1: "State of fear lifted, melted." Getting back in touch with the self that stands behind it all; and increased energy all day. That was very useful in my teaching. Thinking only of the teaching, not thinking about me. Confidence. Self-esteem at least away from rock bottom. Next day start on income tax after long blockage.

"Realising that people do care about me, uncomfortable as I am with that." Energy >, lighter. At a healing centre last night. Lighter. Everything around my eyes was lighter. A fog had lifted.

But then : This morning. Half way back to square one. Completely out of money, and sense of panic about that.
Themes and early circumstances.

My relationship to my father was bad and there are things I regret. I get irritable about stupid things, < morning moods.

Not dealing with things, e.g. never did any homework at home in high school days. The same with auditions. Long standing lack of self-esteem. Background to my life has been guilt, self-criticism, and feeling not at home. When absorbed in something outside myself I get moments of reprieve from this.

When I was three, my mother went to hospital. I've never been much good at staying away. I was put out with other people. Never saw them *(parents)* in three weeks. Not much hanging together in family. When I was five years old I remember a car trip, siblings winding me up. Ashamed at crying, scared that I was lost. Feeling really alone.

07.02.07 *Report. Pl.w 200* last taken 04.02.07

After remedy immediately there is a noticeable strong surge of energy. Then something inside me starts to work against me that wants to fail - wanting the attention and angst. I have spent a lot of my life making myself tired to suppress all this stuff. When I feel connected my self-esteem issue gets into proportion. When I have this increase of energy, I am getting things done that I need to get done. I don't usually multi-task but I brought the typewriter into the kitchen while I was boiling some beans. I am getting on with a lot of stuff – it's a roundabout way of gaining self-esteem. Usually something in me that wants chaos, despair and disillusion destroys the constructive impulses. I do spend a lot of time worried about other people's opinion of me.

15.02.07 Energy reconnecting. Music recording - three days. Energy levels were enough. Not easily happy with the result. When things don't go well get 'attacks from inside' - beating oneself up about the playing - always been there inside my head. All this has buggered up everything I want to do - like driving with the handbrakes on. Came back really tired. Went to healing group. Healing made a huge difference - restored my sanity. Felt more with myself after that - before was beside myself.

Wakes worrying about stuff in middle of the night. Often sleep is disturbed. Just kept control but with awareness: even with problems. Managed to not fall apart and cease to do anything - to take myself in hand. Every aspect of my life is under scrutiny. No use trying to suppress this stuff - things are changing. Examining motivations in things. Why I am doing things? Music etc? Severe confidence problems.

28.02.07 *Took Pl.w 200 yesterday a.m.*
    Has energy, but underneath very tired. Surprised how much energy - but couldn't see straight when looking at music. Attacks re self-esteem but they are not getting through now. Since as long as I can remember, not feeling good about myself: like anti-success gene that wants all this financial crap to happen - likened to a three year old stamping its foot and having a tantrum.
    Overall, still have more energy. Still able to work to a degree. There has been a basic improvement despite what is going on.

21.03.07 *Phone call. Pl.w 200* 09 & 19.03.07. Energy increase each time; handling things with more equanimity and balance.

18.04.07 *Phone call. Took Pl.w 200* 05.04.07. Not taken any more Rx. since. Energy loss has been from lack of sleep and food. Hanging on; > for Rx. re playing in a concert, "Not so wrapped up in my crap". Rx. gives energy. I don't think straight when I get really tired. Getting serious realisations: it doesn't have to be like this. Questions about motivations for playing music - has been a way to be in the world, ego/mind involved. Seeing things more clearly, less from an egotistical point of view.

17.05.07 *Phone call.* I feel changed. No Rx for three weeks now. Gets good patches.
    Re relationship? - always comes away scathed.
    Relationships and work shrinking. Things are coming apart. Entrenched, therefore frightens me. Momentum in certain direction - carrying stuff along. Like the Titanic - needs to be brought to a standstill. Wouldn't turn in time. Waking up and realising who you are. Sadness. Immovability of thing inside.
18.05.07 *Rx: Buddleia 30, 3 in 24 hours.* Good effect.

25.05.07 Able to do things more - paying back bits of owed money. Relationship difficulty - more able to deal with it in a way I would want to.
    Realisation about the thing that happened when I was

three when I was farmed out to another household - three siblings still at home. Always felt out on a limb re siblings. Afraid, ashamed re making a fool of myself, then taunted.

And were there difficult times before you were three ?
I nearly snuffed it *(died)* around my birth.

Looking at the sources of things, I was treated badly by my father. I felt disregarded in respect of being worth anything. Then when he died, the possibility of rapprochement was over. It had not been fulfilled. I have a sense of a past life: the American civil war, two brothers on opposite sides - my father and I. *(He speaks of this with great intensity.)*

After Buddleia 30 : Wants to not be snowed under with anxiety. Instead of being frozen with fear, can pay these people money in bits.

Later this year – October/November – continuing benefits from Buddleia 30 weekly and Plastic wrap 1M every four to six weeks, as required.

Also after Buddleia : "The six weekly doses have had a beneficial accumulative effect – re self-esteem, I can now be impervious to issues without being insensitive to what's goes on; I'm doing what I usually do without the fear, and without the thought that I am not good enough. There have been some bad moments when the strength of this feeling declines, and some big dips too, but the strength still comes out, especially when I am playing music. My aspirations can be grounded by 'the other power' that is destructive. Now I am better able to ignore my habitual devils. Before, I despaired of being able to do anything about it, about those issues that didn't resolve no matter what, despite using various regression treatments.

I realise that I have done so much out of cowardice that I have not been happy with: the inward agenda never matches the outward agenda – dishonesty. I don't think I'm honest with myself or anyone else. When you have played the survival game you're never quite respectable."

I recommend the reader to the Buddleia text in Prometheus No 11 December 1999, and Colin Griffith's The New Materia Medica (Watkins 2007) for further insight into the remedy. (Ed.)

After Plastic wrap : "Before I have been overly deferential to others' thoughts or what they say, wanting everyone to like

me. I'm afraid of disapproval. I wanted approval from my father."
In this feature we can see a connecting link between the two remedies (Ed). For a comparison see Colin Griffith's Buddleia text 'Fear, alienation or hatred felt towards the father figure.'
The New Materia Medica page 148. "I am still procrastinating. If I lack energy it's to do with lack of sleep or food: I'm not my own best friend as far as eating is concerned, but I have more energy after I take the plastic remedy."

CASE 16

Male   34 years old   D.O.B. 23.01.69

M.E. since six years now.

At time of onset, long-term relationship of seven years - with my cousin. Difficult to finish. Abusive emotionally on her part. Three months leading up to it; work frenzy and high impact aerobics and cycling. Draining period. Flu and then when flu lifted, left with fatigue.
Not breast fed. "Not what was done at the time."
13 years old – Glandular fever.
Drugs taken – Cannabis, mostly in teens, occasionally till recently. Speed aged 18/19. Acid three times in early twenties. Last acid trip was scary. Consciousness floating above body – as if it would always be severed.

With M.E. came a loss of confidence re self image as an artist/intellectual. Outer fiction, eloquent, composed individual. I'm OK. Performing self. Desire to rebel against that to be the weakened wreck I feel inside. Wanting to break out of the shell. Wanting to display the vulnerability and appeal for help. Automatic response to lack of attention and lack of warmth from parents. Impacts on relationship with current girlfriend. Present a version of myself - need for love only gets through in little bits.

Pretend to be OK with attacks and what my girlfriend has thrown at me. Take it on board without dealing with it or facing her. Need courage and self-esteem. Self-confidence. Can weather her anger if I would anger. Lack of self-love.

Re cousin - very creative but impaired. Depression. Bulimic. Hid behind her. Deferred my creativity to her's so wouldn't have to risk failure of pushing my stuff into the world. Humiliating sexually in way we made love.

Family history. Mother: highly strung and hysterical; episodes when I was two. Something like a breakdown. Sitting on a shedload of suppressions. I thought, "I'm OK, you don't need to support me, I can do everything by myself."
F. 63. Cancer in last five years. Hodgkin's, throat, chest. Appears to have cleared up.
M. 57. Hysterectomy - irregular periods/heavy flow. High B.P. Diabetic borderline.
"Both are divorced from their bodies and their nature."
MM died - leukaemia. MF died - lung cancer.

Middle child, diplomat, therefore over-polite. Parentage not physically touchy/not emotionally warm, leading to a state where I don't need any warmth as a coping behaviour. Inner sense of frustration/disappointment, rebellion, need. Need to have that support/nourishment. Unfocussed anger. Inner turmoil.

Daily grind of not being able to be creative. Actual physical energy not there to perform songs. Usually caves in after a while. Ambivalence around receiving and asking for warmth. Anxiety about this. Go through fixations about wanting to be free. I have dreams of flying.

Never solid ground on which to make a solid judgement: not sure of awareness of deeper level within me. Lack of response to inner warmth in me.
M.E. - lack of self-belief. Needy and incapable of giving support. Anger sat on. Causing the fatigue. Anger/frustration - blocked anger - shows up in dreams.

When rests in day, images of guns, taking them apart and fiddling with them, this then shifted to bows and arrows - a more empowering positive compulsive image. Compulsive, sexual power and wanting to take it back. Self worth, to gain confidence.

With girlfriend: difficult re no equity. No indulgence or entertainment of my problems.

I feel an intangible weakness in the left side of my body. Not feeling quite right. Less available energy. That side is not as bold or truly there. Sense of imbalance.
14.05.03 *Dream* : Cousin beating me (the abusive relationship). Worst dream I had ever had about her. I was a mess and weep-

ing. My mother came across us fighting and saved me. Afterwards I was in a distraught state and vowed I would never see her again or consent to be anywhere near her. She was coming at me with a battery, very critical of what I was doing. Was it of any value? Mocking of my love for her, especially my physical desires. Me as a man. Value. My desires characterised as aggressive or wrong. She didn't feel I have enough male energy.

Re father. I never sensed he was a strong male presence. Would have liked him to be a stronger and more vibrant character. F not confident with family and intimacy. Fearful about these. F confident in his work in the shop. F - a nothingness there. A vacuum. Nothing negative but no real intimacy/deep affection. As a child, F too distant and M too fragile, therefore created a facade where I didn't need to have expression received. I have no memory of ever being hugged. Mum fear of physicality. Father more prudish.

After Chalcancite 30 2x a week for four weeks. Subtle shifts. Stronger sense of connection to inner self and inner voices - more confidence. More perceptive about issues I need to resolve, the crucial one being the event with my cousin. Sense of surrendering ground around present girlfriend, but stronger sense of my feelings as they happen around her. Shift. Moved from anger and bitterness to feeling wounded. Raw hurt has undermined my confidence and energy. Creativity unsupported by what a sense of stronger family would have given - sense of inadequacy in family history, especially father's side. Confidence that love gives by contact. Need to access depths of my feelings and find sense of purpose.

Lack of intuitive faith. Uncertainty, dread. No understanding of whether anything was good for me. Not linked with myself or life, don't really know what my feelings are doing. Sense of absence. Barrier between me and everyone else - caused by loss of energy that connects mind and body/self with your life. Energy bonds between 'bodies' not there properly.

For information about Chalcancite see Meditative Provings, Madeleine Evans, Rose Press 2000, and Prometheus Journal No 1 1994.

14.08.03 *Dream* : In huge superstore. Continually chased by two terminators - impotent - anger with no focus. Almost escaping.

Every time just avoiding being shot.

Need strength to be honest - sense of connection. Not having barriers of hiding; seeing deeper into yourself and knowing what you are doing. Self-inflicted disappearance. Self-erasure: frightening to behold. Other side is a strong, creative will to express myself in creative terms. I don't feel I have permission to receive love, pleasure, touch; it must always be paid for by giving. If I disappear I will only exist in the other person - re not having sense of deserving to be given to.

Now I feel things: fears/worries. New relationship. Tears. Haven't cried for a long time. Huge emotional release. After release - shocked and shaken by release. This morning very rested; emotionally some space has been freed up.

After Phosphoric acid 6 tds 4/52 - energies improved. Upsurges of grief and weeping from it. Unusual.

Now, as with previous girlfriend, not able to make my voice heard. Feel claustrophobic/trapped emotionally. Obliged to see her when I don't want to. Obliged because otherwise she will feel unattended, not because I am warm/loving. I am frustrated that I don't stand my ground on this matter. Behind is my need to get close and have intimacy/love.

After Pulsatilla 30 : responses to relationship - far more emotional than would usually be. Now more grounded, less fraught and less vulnerable. To do with support - trying to support myself emotionally but not quite having the strength and connectedness to do this. Building a voice, a presence in the world of relationships that is strong and not available to be crushed; built on energy rather than rigidity.

11.03.04 *Remedies: 1) Emerald 30, Thursdays.*
2) Staphisagria 30, Sundays 6/52.

Felt quite a change. Physical sensation which feels good. More direct experience of my physicality, but a lot stirred up in my mind and emotions. More present with pains/experiences. Sense of ambivalence - not really knowing what I feel and what course of action would be best for me. Also a sense of confusion - close to the surface.

Movement towards knowing myself - knowing my inner feelings - strength or self-knowing growing in me.

But still the burden of self-recrimination, being useless

and not going to amount to anything. "Feeling small and unbuilt." Support for some nascent energy and self-knowledge which is there but only a weak flame.

Divorced from inner feelings. Lacking spine/courage to connect with them. Not finding courage to even turn them (feelings) into thoughts. Expectations of others stop me from turning them into action. Struggling to surface and find that will in myself. Compulsive with girlfriend. Trying to manufacture the desire/need to be together.

Fear that drinking the water of knowledge will mean I have to confront people saying that what I want is maybe not what you want. "That's where I have to go. Others will have to lump it." Procrastinating re fear of causing arguments.

Dream : significant re father - extreme necessity to chop off my left hand which was also my father's. No choice but to do it - but in dream never did it. Only lifting blade - plus grief at what a terrible act it would be. *(This recalls the 'intangible' weakness he feels in the left side of his body. Ed)*

Re to let go of aspect of father, re weak role model. Necessity to break from atmosphere of family. Not having faith in my own voice and sense of self. Looking for others' voices to lend authority to mine. Fears of what my girlfriend thinks of me. Will I still be loved if I say what I feel? Ask what she feels first before having a bit of space to say what I feel.

Deeper part of myself hasn't been shown.

Either self sacrifice in relationships or complete separation re not trusting inner voice - lack of connection to deeper intuition. Deeper self neglected - not fully connected up as if mental/emotional presence in my body is very fragile, as if I treat my body like a machine, whatever its state. Body not feeling. To feel more presence in my body, moving towards this. I spend a lot of time around other people in a state of fake consciousness, behaving at being a good person, the one who has no problems. Being unreal. 'Driven from elsewhere.' Secret life where I can be complete; but not allowed to be complete - punishing agency there.

General heaviness, as if unengaged, lack of motivation. Not wanting to be engaged, wanting to side-step, to escape. Lonely feeling, feeling unconnected.

Thirst, great for water and wanting sweet things, ice

cream, fizzy things, citrus, Lemsip etc.

Loss of voice, loss of individuality. Absence. Being there and not there. Sense of loss. Re sense of self and rootlessness. Aloneness, grief. Phantom-like sense of own self-hood. No agency with which to speak, no voice to say what I'm feeling. In my relationship I feel if I had the voice I would say I'm leaving.

14.04.05 *Electricitas 12 bd. 2/52 then Electricitas 18 bd. 4/52.*

Feeling more grounded, less absent both physically and consciousness-wise. Not more available energy but am waking and allowing myself to really be in the world, feel the sensations in my body and not feeling depressed or victimised by them. Not overwhelmed by tension - its more fluid - not so fixed. Feel quite erratic about the way I feel about myself - e.g. that I am worthless, socially inept, as if personality at zero, failure, generating out of nothing, no presence, status, worry about my future; or I enjoy the sunshine and feel all right.

Even before the M.E. - no foundation: inadequacy re not touched/nurtured or given palpable sense of self-confidence, therefore felt more stupid than others and 'would take longer to get there.' Vulnerable creative side, want to create more, (as if other people are not going to be derisory,) but not able to. Creative, artistic, being an outsider, feeling of worthlessness - fear of people - being seen by others. Need to be close to people - also to hold them at arm's length.

Re guitar making course, internalised, abstract ideas, intellectual. Grounding, wood and sound - physical. I feel moved to be so close to this truth. I want to have the energy to do it.

Electrcitas 30 daily.

Dream of vulnerability, relationships and longing for closeness. Dreams of victim-hood, betrayed, let down. Sitting on a lot of feelings inacted on, feelings now there – closer than used to be; not in touch/too cowardly to let them in. If lets them in would become selfish - not attractive, will hurt people. I want to be myself and not worry about what others think of me.

Calcarea sulphuricum 30 bd 10/7.

Relationship with F is better than it was, generally more accepting and neutral around family. *Since Calc. Sulph.* less conscious of those feelings of what others think, happier with that aspect of my personality.

Digitalis 12 tds 5/7 re heart palpitations, symptoms of long standing. Heart feels drained, exhausted.

After Dig. 12 more heavy in a connected way. Grounded on planet earth. Seeing things more vividly. "So much in my own mind, it's not often that I land on terra firma." No easy link between me and other people - it doesn't flow, as if they are alien. Fragmented, broken up, disjuncture within myself. Always intellectualising stuff.

Feeling outside of social world; I do not have fully fledged self, fragmented, living in a state of silence. Feel self to be out there in the silence. Learnt a performance of language - not natural. Sense of isolation exacerbated by M.E. because forced away from society - is this a desire? I like to be in my own cocoon - comfortable. As a child, learnt script of comedies to be part of gang - had to make up for shortfall in self. As teenager, not part of group – did not feel it. Vulnerable, challenged. Not comfortable, not relaxed in relationships and groups.

Now, in relationships it feels difficult to communicate; I worry about being too quiet. Not wanting to talk but feel should. Self sufficient but not with grounding or strength.

09.03.07 *Plastic wrap 30, weekly 4/52.*

Dream, during these weeks: Cut own fingers off - realise - cry - try to put them back on.

10.05.07. *Pl.w. - after fourth dose.* "Most profound physical effect of any remedy that I have had." Top of left shoulder - looked like insect bites. Red, swollen, painful and sore and itchy. Two days later, soreness and tenderness, down arm and to breast area. Doctor said, "Looks like shingles." Pains in arms constant, < night. Swelling down now. Since swelling calmed down, have been feeling emotional anxiety. More grounded, more emotional, more able to feel my emotions, and allow myself to feel them. I have been so internalised, and so my contact with the outside world has been tenuous. It is as if there are ways of being I may not be able to experience: an intuitive connection with world.

One morning driving along, swathe of emotion - panic, grief. Stomach goes cold and sudden emotional/bodily realisation of the trouble you are in - like might be pulled over by the police, or stopped for a crime. Felt at point of stopping car. This was all triggered by listening to a song: the song was inscrutable - can penetrate from different angles but not reach to centre. Trapped in an internalised state. Powerful emotion that I know was pure - not filtered by any intellectualisation.

At this time an awakening of connection with his emotions, also reconnecting with the world of nature with a new interest in gardening. These were clear indications of the benefits of this remedy for him. Other remedies were of value after this but he never looked back in this respect. (Ed.)

The following two dreams were during this time :
29.03.07 *Dream of a boat.* I was on some kind of boat; we had been warned that it was dangerous, that there might be some kind of accident. I saw a huge sailboat spinning towards us across the water, like it was a spinning top. I was the first to see it and I told everyone what I saw. We were told that we should all go to the back of the boat, which was just like a floating building. So I went to the back with my sister, we got there and I said grab onto this life raft, and if the boat hits, we'll jump into the water and inflate the life raft and help others onto it. I looked around and my sister was already in the water floating away. I was scared, so I pushed myself into the water as well, pushing the life raft towards her, in fact I grabbed a lifejacket, which was huge, and threw it to her and told her to inflate it, which she did. Then I swam towards another person who was floating on a large canoe that looked like a coffin. I saw lots of people in the water, survivors from the other boats. I managed to pull myself and my sister onto the coffin/canoe, and then my parents were nearby, my sister went with them. I sat on top of this person, laid out on the coffin/canoe, and kept this person company with inane, keep-your-spirits-up chit-chat, though I didn't know if they were alive or dead.
27.04.07 *Dream :* I was both watching and taking part in a TV program. Within minutes of arriving in a strange place, they (director and assistant) discover there is a solitary Dalek in the centre of the town. It fires at the director. The town is in a central valley, with cliffs and hills surrounding it. To begin with I am the director's assistant, but then I become a character who's been there a long time. She is a feral outcast who is pitied by the townfolk, but who somehow has been driven mad by the presence of the Dalek, and has become a sort of 'Tom of Bedlam' character

(though I think she's female), who is seen as mad but harmless by the townspeople. Somehow she's also in a secret cult to do with suicide, which comprises just three or four women in the town. There's a long chase sequence between her and the director and his assistant. I am too cunning and have planned too well to be caught. I hide beneath a bush, am discovered, but then I have an escape route, a vine to swing to another cliff, and it takes a long time for the director to catch up with me. Each time they catch up with me, I elude them. I'm naked from the waist up, a green skirt beneath, scars on my back, knotted matted hair. I'm pleased to be so free of social convention, though I am lonely. I am somehow destined to kill the Dalek, the evil in our midst, though I don't know how.

Compare with the Catskin-type tales in The Cinderella Connection. Page 187.

Energy levels? Waking feeling little bit of energy but not a lot. Cloudy in my mind.

I do feel able to allow my emotions without them being doctored by my intellect. Spontaneous feeling of love for girl-friend. Trust. Direct feeling of the moment. Some essential part of me is shut off from world of society. More aware of that. As if existing independently – a parallel world. This is mostly the case, girlfriend as the exception. 'Losing your mind is coming through to a state of feeling.' Every small operation I have to decide on. Enjoying going out in garden and doing things in it. First time ever. Since first Plastic. Want to adjust to natural rhythm – to get to sleep earlier.

I ask about his feelings. Outside calm, Mr Perfect. Inside conflict and rebellion against calm exterior – it's 'not done' to show feelings – stressed, frustrated.

03.07.07 *Dream* : I was sleeping outside in a big field. As I woke up I thought I was alone, but as I rolled over I could feel some-one or something else under the plastic sheet I was on. The thing was sharp beneath me, like rose thorns or bramble. I rolled off it to find out if it was something alive, and it moved. I grabbed it, bravely, and it struggled. I held on, it was very sharp, digging into my hands. I struggled to wake up more, but kept my hold. I pulled the plastic away and saw it was my sister. She looked just ordinary, but there were knives coming out of her arms, and even larger knives coming out of her feet, that had pierced her legs and were digging into me. I held her, she seemed upset, sick somehow. I held her more, and when I could I picked her up; she was quite heavy, and suddenly her boyfriend was here. We carried her through a corridor (we were inside now) into my Mum and Dad's room, and I lay her on the bed. My Mum and Dad were getting ready for bed, but not yet in bed. My sister still had knives coming out of her. As I put her down, her head was a strange shape. She was on her back with her knees up, unable to straighten her legs. I could see a terribly sharp set of scissors coming out of her head. She was in a strange state of rigor mortis, or paralysis. Her head started to swell, I could see she was terrified, and all she said was, "I'm dead". I said reassuringly, "You're not dead, you're ill", and I looked at my Mum and expected them to take her to hospital. I didn't know what to say. I woke up and had to put the light on, I was upset.

Reflecting on the dream : My sister is five years younger than me, someone I care about; but in the dream it is dangerous to be close to her. She is energetic, fun-loving and sociable – I have been closer to her for longer than with anyone else, e.g. holding her hand when walking out.

Knives - doing her harm. Conflicting parts of myself.

Knives symbolising seizure/attack.

That the dream was outdoors connects with a feeling of being somehow complete. This reflects the closer relation I now have with my inner feelings and nature.

05.07.07 *Pl.w 1M to take weekly for nine weeks.*

After taking the first tablet in the session - relaxation down sides, sinking moving down, relaxing into my body. Head connecting with my body. Neck pain - this passes soon. Relaxing now up to top of head. Light seems less harsh in my eyes.

Phone report two weeks later : Once, on taking the weekly tablet, I felt light-headed; another time I felt 'grounded' with a sense of energy moving down through body.

Thumb knuckle, left hand and weakness in left arm. Arthritis signs? Down forearm. Same arm as had shingles on shoulder.

Energy-wise not much to report - much the same.

08.09.07 *Dream* : Trying to keep door closed in respect of stranger coming in. Either restrained/paralysed despite trying to move arm - Herculean effort. Dream set in flat, everyday. *(Dreams now of the present time; before they were either of the past or abstracted.)* Trying to move while still asleep. Impotence of will against state of paralysis.

Re feelings with girlfriend – have felt a sense of connection - part of me feeling more within myself rather than beside myself. Physical contact more vibrant, less fearful. Less bound, guarded and reserved. Noticed this in last two or three weeks especially. Difficult to imagine my own person-hood distinctly, therefore guarded. Such a thin membrane, open to influence. Openness, therefore guarded.

Dreams : Self-harm; suicide; knives; bodily paralysis; harm to family.

Melancholic streak - suicide as symbolic of this sadness. Knives as expression of frustration and anger at not giving more time to myself. Doing duty even although doesn't want to. Anger re feelings of powerlessness turned into an image of power and revenge.

Repeated image: dead rabbit held by its feet.

Sequential image: gun at my head, sword-person wielding a sword. Archery - fixing an arrow - seeing arrow in flight.

His review a year later

07.11.08 Thoughts on the Plastic wrap remedy, and how I feel now.

"I had been seeing my homoeopath regularly for several years before taking the Plastic wrap remedy. On many occasions, I had described feelings of isolation both from myself, from the world of people, and from the physical or 'natural' world. I felt that my sense of self was provisional, fragmented, holding together only by the weakest of bonds. This made me feel vulnerable to the demands and expectations of others, and as if I would disintegrate into the stronger personalities around me. I also felt unable to access most of my deeper emotional self, so that understanding or articulating my feelings was very hard, as I only had fleeting glimpses of what they were.

After taking the Plastic wrap, I had several dreams and

experiences that put me directly in touch with a deeper emotional sense of myself. The most profound of these happened whilst I was driving in my car, listening to a song that seemed to speak to me on a mysterious level that, although I could not grasp it rationally, gave me an almost overwhelming feeling of grief and sadness that felt at the same time liberating and strangely significant. Since then, although I cannot say I have resolved or understood my insecurities, I do feel them in a more tangible, visceral way. I have since this time also taken up some gentle gardening, which I find very enjoyable and nourishing. I feel grounded when I garden, and have become more aware of the seasons and the natural, physical world around me.

I recently had a dream (7th Oct '08), vivid and brief, that kept my mind busy for the remainder of that night, and that seemed highly significant. I wrote it down at the time like this:

> coming home as usual
> with friends who find it natural
> to cross this membrane between worlds
> where the grass glistening underfoot
> switches over in an instant
> to a roof of shimmering stars
> dizzying overhead, to which i
> never find it easy to adjust

In the dream it was night, pleasant and warm, with stars overhead and moonlight setting the dewy grass glimmering. I was with friends, on the way home from an evening out. At a certain point on a grassy slope, we had to pass through some kind of invisible threshold, beyond which the world was flipped upside down. While my friends were used to this, I found it difficult to make the transition, and for some moments I felt dizzy and disoriented, as my feet seemed to be walking on the stars, and the glistening grass was overhead. It took an act of will and imagination for me to accept this as the new normality, which I did manage.

In discussion with my homoeopath the day after this dream, some possible meanings emerged. I realised that two recent bursts of confidence and pleasure in the company of others had come as a surprise to me. These both occurred at birthday parties of friends at which I led a fun sing-along to popular tunes on my acoustic guitar. I was surprised at how much I enjoyed singing in company, and how relaxed and uninhibited I became, even though a lot of attention was on me. Thinking of this, and some other related moments, is still surprising for me, and a little disorienting, as if a new way of thinking about myself has arisen – a new model of selfhood, without the vulnerability and smallness – which seems unfamiliar and a little frightening. It feels as if I must use my will and imagination to keep hold of this new sense of myself, and that it will take time for it become familiar and 'normal'. This dizzying upside-down flip in the dream may link to this new confidence, it being so radically different to my usual discomfort in company, so that although it was a good experience, it felt as strange as the world turning on its head.

The soft, kindly imagery of nature in the dream also seemed meaningful. In quite a few earlier dreams, animals in particular were hostile and attacking, and the landscape itself was often harsh, phantasmagoric and even apocalyptic, with earthquakes crumbling the ground beneath my feet. In this dream, though, the grassland was soft and rolling, the air balmy, the starlight beautiful. This links quite strongly, I think, to my new-found pleasure in gardening, and more importantly, perhaps, to the more vital connection I feel to my deeper feelings, to the emotional 'ground' of my unconscious life."

2009 - Conium followed well; and later on Calcarea Carbonica as well as Pl.w 10M.

CHAPTER EIGHT

Meditative 'provings' of 1997

These are the notes from each of the thirteen partici-
pants. They 'received' their information independently, by holding
a tablet in their hand. This was not done as a group.

*Italics (for features that appear elsewhere in this book) are
mine. SD Ed.*

1) The 6 C potency: The first thing that occurs to me as I open
the packet, is something to do with the *stomach*, and then it's
to do with *pregnancy*, or a sense of softness, and I see pink. I'm
holding the tablet now. My first image is of *water*. It feels - if
you imagine *two poles of extremes - then this is sort of in the
middle*. It's a bit stodgy, it's fairly dense; it's either something
that lightens the dense condition, or it's the other way round -
that *it's something that brings together.* It feels *calming,* soothing, bringing together. But I guess all remedies do that . . . God
knows what I'm in at the moment! - *I'm so spaced out!* It feels
quite serious . . . *It's a bit stuck.* Yes, it's a very definite picture
- something to do with calming keeps coming up. Something like
hard-headed, and I would say that it has some sort of dense
physical symptoms, maybe blockages, or like a sense of hardening
- like constipation, or possibly headache. It's like having a cloud
around you or within you, and it's grey. It's to do with thinking
too, thinking patterns are quite slow, stubborn and unchangeable.
It's a bit depressed actually. *It's a stuck feeling, like I'm used to
it, or can't, or I almost don't want to change, even though I know
this isn't working.*

The 30 C potency: I'm holding the 30 C potency now. I'm
getting a funny feeling in my head now - sinuses. I can feel
something happening all the way from the forehead over the
head to the neck, like I'm getting a cold. It's a tightness. It
makes me want to screw up my eyes. It's like if you had something like a dog, or fur, or wool and initially it's matted together
and the remedy somehow combs it out. *It lightens up.*

Now a mild sense of *panic*, to do with the feeling of letting go of previous structures. It is about change, opening rather than being not so much closed as densely bunched together, out of habit. This is a feeling of dissolving, but also of *opening and revealing.* So new insecurities come in because it reveals the vulnerability that the holding was trying to protect against.

Now about the physical body - a sense of sickness, or *nausea, or fear in the stomach, or travel sickness, or morning sickness* even. I don't know if this is a remedy to avoid in pregnancy or it would be good in *pregnancy.* Intellectually, I'd say it maybe is a bit much in pregnancy unless opening is welcomed. It's a sense of having to trust as well. If other support systems are not there, this may make you too open. It's feeling the need to defend, or a slight fear. It does also have a soothing quality. It's a powerful feeling. It's not like a soft cotton wool blanket soothe. *It's a "Come on, grow up, face things" or "You can do it" sort of soothe.* I sense that this would work very well with some other remedy, to give really solid support on another level. This again may be just how it's affecting me, because there's a feeling of "Am I ready to feel safe in this?" *It's like opening out a certain amount, and if the real safety isn't there, I want to pull myself in again, but I can't.* I can't access the same patterns to pull in because it has melted them; so if it was someone who is able to acknowledge that their life isn't working, or their responses aren't working, if they were able to say, "I want to let go and I can't" - then it feels like a gentle and powerful way to do that. It facilitates that. But if they are hanging on for dear life, then it feels like there's another thing needed, something more.

The 6 C potency again: I'm finding this is making me quite *woozy.* It has a layer to do with shock, a feeling of shock. It soothes it, but it doesn't take it away, it just *prepares the ground for something else.*

30 C again: If someone was already feeling quite open, or on the verge of tears, maybe it would expand that and give release, or it breaks the hold, so that things start to move. I'm getting the intestines image again. If there is dense matter packed in the intestines, this would be a subtle and gentle relaxant. It doesn't necessarily break up the matter, at least not at this potency (the 30 C). It relaxes the muscle walls so the intestines themselves soften. I still get this feeling of *opening.*

Also that this works in partnership with something else, or with two something elses, depending on what the desired effects are, but something else that acts with this action. I think this may also be good for children, just a hunch. It's quite gentle and subtle, but it's quite strong. It's about trust and letting go of control. But letting go of control requires trust, otherwise it feels out of control and creates contraction to try and stop the process. And this definitely doesn't make contraction of this sort very easy. If you had someone very uptight who wasn't trusting when the support was there for them and who had some circulation or bowel thing, then it would be very interesting to see how it would work out for them.

2) Awareness of heart centre - tugging or tightness. Relaxing of top of arms - heaviness. Hot vulva. Jitteriness as after strong coffee. *Wondering if it is an aphrodisiac, but no lascivious thoughts. Dry mouth. Relaxation, calmness.* 'Thick head', a bit like when ill in bed as a child, sense of unreality. Tingling skin on cheeks.

3) Meditation. I saw a large pink area. I saw a slow burning fire with grey embers as if of burning wood. I then saw a large green area and thought, "That's a nice lawn". Then I saw two large molluscs, slug type things with feelers at the front, and they were side by side on top of a small waterfall, but without danger of the fast water throwing them over as they were lodged on the shallow rocks. I then saw the underside of one of them. It had glowing parts underneath. I then saw a mechanical screw or worm in a red box.

4) Initially almost tearful, quickly followed by being contented. Indigestion. Saw a lot of purple and *blue, green* later on. *Warmth, calmness.* My place in *nature* kept changing - I started off on a grassy hill with a lake, willow trees, swans, and lots of bright flowers, then I was on a windswept beach! Then sunflowers predominantly, seen on their own. They kept flashing into my mind.

5) Took myself off into a field of buttercups which I would never do in meditation. Usually I would pick a tree near a stream. Only physical symptom I noticed was my eyelids felt jumpy.

6) Initially the smell of disinfectant. Feeling of great coldness (I was told this would be in the context of fever and heat), particularly felt in the head. Pain in top left part of my head, heavy, clamped feeling, top of head. Feeling of numbness, coldness in neck (base of head) followed by pain in root of nose, extending down nose and out to cheeks. Left nostril, wanting to sneeze. Face felt as if lots of small tremors taking place. Cold. *Heavy swashing feeling in legs. Thoughts of the sea.* Tickle in throat. Dry. Heart seemed to alter rhythm slightly, slower and heavier. Pain in left breast. *Slight feeling of nausea. Feeling of depression, apathy, helplessness.* Stiffness in face. Tremors back of neck. Sudden itching between eyebrows.

7) *Peaceful.* Cleansing. Yellow flower? Dandelion? Green leaves. Lungs? Liver-detoxifying. Purifying the blood. Digestion - aids digestion. Floating spots in front of eyes. Urinary system, copious urination? General feeling of > *for fresh air,* > for sunshine. *Calming in the Solar plexus.*

8) My son showed me a mushroom/toadstool. Shortly after holding remedy, a burning sensation in the palm of my hand. Then a short lasting pain lower back, left side. Feeling of slight soreness left side of throat. Slight headache above left eyebrow. Nerve twitching inner side of left thigh. Right wrist and part of hand itchy. Itchy left eyebrow, like < wool. Slight pain in outer side of right breast towards armpit and down into inner side of upper arm. Tingling in nose - irritation. *Itchiness increased and moving to various parts of body - legs/face.*

9) Immediately upon touching remedy I was transformed to the beach. *A very balancing effect, grounded, feet very firmly standing, balanced. A feeling of calmness: non-hurried. A feeling of being balanced within the inner body.* A need to be calm and listen, an eagerness to listen and learn. Looking at the yellow sand. A need to stay rooted, not to move on - here and now - to stay in the moment, to stand and listen and watch. A desire to look in to the land, no desire to look at the water or out to sea - only to look inland, steady; saw movements away from the water towards the land. *Very grounding.* Wanting to stay and move very slowly. > wind, especially blowing from the sea into land. *No anxiety, and*

appetite better. > *Fresh air.* A mild deep-acting, *balancing remedy.* A desire to stay, listen and take on board. Non-hurried.

10) Felt tingling in hand that held remedy, for a few minutes. I was on a grassy bank under a tree with a view of the sea. *(The natural world and water, again. Ed.)* Heard sea crashing on shore. A woman came to tell me about the remedy. Saw a sunflower, then I thought of 'heartsease.' Saw a violet/blue colour. I felt relaxed, quite calm, but had a slight headache at front of head. Hand holding remedy felt very slightly warmer.

11) Physical sensations: Heat of hand holding the remedy, delicious feeling of warmth in solar plexus. Impressions/Ideas: Constriction of heart. Old hurt/pain. Tears. The same feeling of constriction of heart came up several times. Burning lips?

12) Totally relaxed. Sleepy, contented and warm. As if someone was pressing down on my right finger initially. No other physical symptoms, except sleepiness.

13) A child scratching/tearing at its upper arms - eczema, crying with pain. Headache, - inside to frontal. Heavy. Dry, rawness of throat < swallowing. Tightness around sternum, *slight difficulty breathing*. I couldn't end the session, I felt tired, hopeless, sad. I couldn't rouse myself to speak, it suddenly seemed pointless. I am left with a heavy heart and upper chest - more emotional than physical. I feel drained of emotional energy, too many steps to reach any goal. I feel sad, not smiling any more. I feel paralysed, a weak feeling, but I know I could do what I have to do - but can't rouse myself. Sighing. Weakness, arms, from shoulders. Later, deep pain, upper, inner corner of right scapula. A remedy of inflammation and despair.

CHAPTER NINE

The Cinderella Connection.

Beauty, truth, and rarity
Grace in all simplicity,
Here enclosed in cinders lie.

I have noticed several parallels between themes that arise in both the proving and cases of Plastic wrap and Cinderella type stories. The 'fairy tale' appears in many different guises, from ancient China to contemporary reworkings in films. In Britain the best known version is from the French tradition as written down by Perrault in 1697. This is the one with the fairy God-(good) mother by whom a pumpkin is transformed into a golden carriage etc.

First of all, and in some detail, I will give extracts from the Germanic version in the Grimm brothers' collection of fairy tales published in 1812, and make comparisons with the proving and some case examples.

Themes are in Bold; *extracts from the Grimm text are in italics.*

The first and 'good' mother. *The wife of a rich man fell sick, and as she felt that her end was drawing near, she called her only daughter to her bedside and said: 'Dear child, be good and pious, and then the good God will always protect you, and I will look down on you from heaven and be near you.' Thereupon she closed her eyes and departed. Every day the maiden went out to her mother's grave and wept, and she remained pious and good.*
Compare : prover no. seven's concluding review, page 77.

The father takes another wife, the 'wicked' stepmother; she has her own daughters. *The woman had brought with her into the house two daughters, who were beautiful and fair of face, but vile and black of heart. Now began a bad time for the poor stepchild.*

Cinderella's mother has died. She is no longer with her own mother and her father does not protect her. She faces great difficulties in this new domestic set-up.

Compare :

Case 8. Her mother is absorbed and pre-occupied by a state of self-pity and blame; her father has been completely absent since the very beginning of her life. She has difficulties with her sister as well, is troubled by a sense of 'having no family'.

Case 9. She has had to 'find her own voice' in relation to her mother.

Case 10. Parents split up, mother gone, then left to her own devices by her father as well. Extreme difficulties with siblings.

Case 11. Father and mother split up when she was five. Father not much present after this.

Case 12. Not understood by parents, poor relationship with mother especially. Mother absent when she was a young child.

Clothing and footwear. *They took her pretty clothes away from her, put an old grey bed gown on her, and gave her wooden shoes.*

The theme of clothing - dress and footwear, begins here; grey and heavy, compared to her previous and familiar pretty clothes.

Mocked for her appearance. *'Just look at the proud princess, how decked out she is!' they cried, and laughed and led her into the kitchen.*

The ashes. *In the evening when she had worked till she was weary she had nowhere to go, but had to sleep by the hearth in the cinders.*

Compare here Robert Bly's book Iron John, first published in 1990; this is a version of the story first known as Iron Hans, which also appears in the Grimm's collection. In the chapter 'The Road of the Ashes, Descent and Grief' he offers a wide-ranging discussion and analysis of the theme which he calls 'Descent to the ashes.' The directly relevant sections are : Taking Kitchen Work, Katabasis, and Taking the Road of the Ashes. The following extract comes from the last of these three sections.

"'Ashes" and "cinders" in fairy tales are code words for the ashy, sooty, depressed, "out of it" time. We imagine in our day that to be assigned to the hearth is some sort of punishment, but in the fairy stories that assignment goes to the lucky third son, who is the magical ashy fool, and to the lucky third daughter, Cinderella, the magical suffering child of the mother. For those two children, tending the hearth is the right task.'

Back again to the Cinderella story:
Artifice, fine clothing and jewellery vis-à-vis the natural and supernatural worlds. Trees, water and wells. *It happened that the father was once going to the fair, and he asked his two stepdaughters what he should bring back for them. 'Beautiful dresses,' said one, 'Pearls and jewels,' said the second. 'And you, Cinderella,' said he, 'What will you have?' 'Father, break off for me the first branch which knocks against your hat on your way home.'*

Plastic wrap may be a useful remedy for those who are preoccupied with their appearance in ways that place artificial above natural beauty. Consider image-conscious teenagers, girls especially, and also eight to twelve year olds.
Case 8. Referring to her family sense of image : 'It was all about impression and not real.'

When he reached home he gave his stepdaughters the things which they had wished for, and to Cinderella he gave the branch from the hazel bush which had brushed against him on his way home and knocked off his hat.

In 19th century Germany it was thought that there were witches beneath the bark of hazel trees. Forked hazel twigs are used for divining rods. Hazels assist the power of magic spells. For the Celts they were magic trees that produce flowers and fruits, beauty and wisdom at the same time. They considered it to be a 'Tree of Knowledge.' The wisdom of the hazel is not the wisdom of great age and experience, but that of simplicity and innocence. The tree is associated with knowledge, creativity and magical powers. (From The Living Wisdom of Trees by Fred Hageneder.)

Magical uses of hazel (from Tree Medicine, Tree Magic by Ellen Evert Hopman) : 'Hazel trees bestow fertility, protection and wisdom. Wear a hazel crown to strengthen wish manifestation. In England the hazelnut was used for love divination on Halloween. The hazel tree was venerated by the ancient Celts for having a special association with sacred springs and wells. To the Celts, water was seen as the entrance to the Otherworld and offerings could be made to the Gods by dropping hazelnuts into lakes and wells.'

See also the 'Sensations relating to water' section in the proving, especially the dreams. (Page number 29). In other versions of the Cinderella-type story pools of water or wells are important.

Wishes granted in a supernatural way via the world of nature.

Cinderella went to her mother's grave and planted the hazel branch on it, and wept so much that the tears fell down on it and watered it. Thrice a day Cinderella went and sat beneath it, and wept and prayed, and a little white bird always came on the tree, and if Cinderella expressed a wish, the bird threw down to her what she had wished for.

In other versions wishes are granted by an animal; a cow or a fish for example.

Male-female relationship and courtship.

Up to this point in the tale we have been introduced to Cinderella in the context of her mother, now dead, and her father. Also we have seen her in relationship with a step mother and sisters. Next a King and his son come into the story. The King's son is to choose a bride.

It happened, however, that the King gave orders for a festival which was to last three days, and to which all the beautiful young girls in the country were invited, in order that his son might choose himself a bride.

The two stepsisters prepare themselves.

Cinderella would have liked to go with them to the dance, and begged her step-mother to allow her to do so. "You go, Cinderella!" said she; "covered in dust and dirt as you are, and would go to the festival? You have no clothes and shoes, and yet would dance!"

(See prover number seven's supervisor's story of going clubbing! Page 80.)

She is given increasingly difficult 'impossible' tasks by the step-mother. She goes into the garden and calls to pigeons and turtle-doves and 'all the birds beneath the sky' to come and help her with the tasks; but, despite completing them in time, the step-mother says: *No, Cinderella, you have no clothes and you cannot dance: you would only be laughed at, and we would be ashamed of you!* And off she goes with her two daughters to the festival.

As no one was now at home, Cinderella went to her mother's grave beneath the hazel tree, and cried: 'Shiver and quiver, little tree, Silver and gold throw down over me.' Then the bird threw a gold and silver dress down to her, and slippers embroidered with silk and silver. She put on the dress with all speed, and went to the festival.
Compare Case 8: her dream of being at a party wearing glittery, silver dance shoes (page 115).

The prince approached her, took her by the hand and danced with her. He would dance with no other maiden, and never let loose of her hand, and if anyone else came to invite her, he said: "This is my partner."
Cinderella is brought to a position equal to the King's son.
Compare Case 9 again: she finds herself in a new kind of equality in relationship after first taking Plastic wrap (page 114).

She danced till it was evening, and then she wanted to go home. Two evenings in succession she goes to dance and each time at the end of the evening she escapes from the prince.

On the third evening *the King's son, however, had employed a ruse, and had caused the whole staircase to be smeared with pitch, and there, when she ran down, had the maiden's left slipper remained stuck. The King's son picked it up, and it was small and dainty, and all golden. Next morning, he went with it to the father, and said to him: "No one shall be my wife but she whose foot this golden slipper fits."*

When the two sisters each try on the slipper it is too small; but, encouraged by their mother - *"When you are Queen you will have no more need to go on foot"* - one of them cuts a toe off and then the other slices off a bit of her heel to force their foot into the shoe.
See Case 10 (cutting her feet) and Prover 10's supervisor's note.

The prince rides off with one and then the other and each

time the pigeons in the hazel tree call out to him as he passes:
'Turn and peep, turn and peep, There's blood within the shoe,
The shoe is too small for her, The true bride waits for you.'

Cinderella is brought to the King's son. *Then she seated herself on a stool, drew her foot out of the heavy wooden shoe, and put it into the slipper, which fitted like a glove.*

Compare here the 'Precise detail' section in the proving (page 15). Also my note on 'Precision and exactness' (page 84).

And when she rose up and the King's son looked at her face he recognized the beautiful maiden who had danced with him and cried: "That is the true bride!"

He takes Cinderella on his horse and rides away with her. They pass by the hazel tree – the two white doves *came flying down and placed themselves on Cinderella's shoulders, one on the right, the other on the left, and remained sitting there.*

The tree and the birds associated with her mother's grave. confirm the outcome: the white doves as a symbol of her protection and natural purity?

Other versions considered

In the 1890's Marian Roalfe compiled a collection entitled '345 Variants of the Cinderella Story.' She writes that, as a type, they are stories of 'person in a mean or obscure position who, by means of supernatural assistance, makes a good marriage.' This sequence is enriched by incidents, typically including an unkind stepmother, jealous sisters, the eventual recognition by the exact fitting of a shoe or ring, or a matching lock of hair *(c.f. the story of Tristan and Isolde)*, and the hostile persons forgiven or punished. In the most archaic versions the dead mother 'returns' in the form of beast or animal to reveal the magical means that can help the child through its ordeals.

She identifies three types : A) Cinderella. The ill-treated heroine and the recognition by means of a shoe. B) Catskin. The 'unnatural' father who pays his daughter inappropriate attention. Heroine flight. Donkeyskin-type stories are also part of this group. C) Cap o'Rushes. King Lear judgement. Outcast heroine.

She lists the themes : Aid. Animal witness. Countertasks. Dead father help. Dead (or transformed) mother help. Eating taboo. False bride. Happy marriage. Heath abode (in a wild inhospitable place). Help at grave. Helpful animal. Heroine or hero disguise and flight. Hiding box. Ill-treated heroine or hero. Lost shoe. Lovesick prince. Magic dresses. Marriage tests. Meeting-place. Menial heroine or hero. Mutilated feet. Outcast heroine and hero. Pitch (tar) trap. Recognition by means of shoe or ring. Revivified bones. Shoe marriage test. Slaying of the helpful animal. Substituted bride (unsuccessful in the end). Surprise rencontre. Tasks. Task-performing animal. Threefold flight. Token objects. Villain nemesis.

The earliest datable version of the Cinderella type of story anywhere in the world occurs in a Chinese book written about 850-860 AD.

It goes like this: A man marries two wives. One dies. She has a daughter called Yeh-Hsien, intelligent and good at making pottery. Her father loves her. He then dies and she is ill-treated by the step mother; made to work for her, collecting firewood in dangerous places and drawing water from deep pools. She gets a small fish with red fins and golden eyes and puts it in a bowl of water. As it grows bigger she finds larger bowls for it and eventually she puts it into the pond. 'When she came to the pond, the fish always exposed its head and pillowed it on the bank; but when anyone else came, it did not come out.' Jealous of this the step mother by deception attracts the fish out of the pond and kills it. She cooks it and serves it up. 'It tasted twice as good as an ordinary fish.' The bones are hidden under a dung heap. Yeh-hsien is then directed by a man appearing to her in the sky to get the fish bones and hide them in her room.

She is told that the fish's bones are magical: 'Whatever you want, you have only to pray to them for it.' She is now able to provide herself with gold, pearls, dresses and food whenever she wants them. So she can then go, unbeknown to her step mother, to the Cave Festival. 'This is a ceremony of ancestor worship and at the same time a mating festival.' She wears a cloak spun from kingfisher feathers and shoes of gold. The step mother, who is also at the festival, suspects something so Yeh-hsien leaves, but in such a hurry that she loses one of the golden shoes. In the end the shoe reaches the King who lives on an island. All the women in the kingdom try it on and there is not one that it fits. Eventually he finds Yeh-Hsien. The shoe fits her. She crosses the sea to be his chief wife.

(From Arthur Waley: The Chinese Cinderella Story, in the journal Folklore No 58, 1947.)

Themes from these and other versions.

The silk (or pearl or copper) to silver, then gold sequence.

In some versions of the story, the heroine goes to the dancing the first time wearing silver shoes, and the next night golden shoes. As I understand it, silver can stand symbolically for the Moon/female energy archetype, and gold for the Sun/male side. In other examples the sequence starts with silk, pearl or copper before the silver and gold. Copper is associated with Venus/Cyprus/Cupros.

In the Donkeyskin type the threefold magical dress sequence is: the colour of the seasons, the night sky, with moon and stars, then the colour of the sun, made of gold and diamonds.

Shoes as symbols. (From The Element Encyclopaedia of Symbols.)

Shoes. 'Freudians regard them as phallic, Diel views them as the symbol of the soul – a point of contact between the body and the earth, a symbol of the principle of reality: "He has his feet on the ground."

In antiquity, the wearing of shoes was the privelege and symbol of a free man and his power; slaves went barefoot.

In addition, the shoe (which has a female form, as it were) is related to the symbolic phallic significance of the foot and was a fertility symbol in various harvest and wedding customs.' See Editor's dream no 7 (page 83).

There are also *Token objects – Towel – Comb – Water,* the water as mirror. In one example they look in the well to see which of them is the more beautiful – Beauty or Pock Face, the cruel daughter of the second wife.

In one Catskin type story, the father wanted a boy. A girl is born, and then disowned by the father. The girl wears a series of different clothes: a coat of silver cloth, the next of beaten gold, then one made of all the feathers of all the birds of the air. Finally, to make her canny and necessary escape, she dons a catskin. At the ball, when it came to parting time, the young lord said, "Pray tell me, fair maid, where you live." But Catskin curtsied and said "Kind sir, if the truth I must tell, At the sign of the 'Basin of water' I dwell." Compare again with the 'Sensations relating to water' in the Mind section of the proving text (page 29).

Consideration of the views of some other commentators.

Several commentators have written about the various versions. Jack Zipes takes a socio-political view in his book 'The Brothers Grimm'. He describes how these tales have evolved, over four thousand years, reflecting changes in society. The earliest types describe a resourceful young woman pursuing her own destiny guided by a wise, gift-bearing but recently deceased mother. These are oral tales celebrating the ritualistic initiation of a girl entering womanhood. In an early Iranian version he sees an affinity to matrilineal moon worship. Then the 1634 Italian version 'The Cat Cinderella' reflects what he calls patrialisation. Here a governess is demonised, the heroine is domesticated before she can marry, and then she is rescued by a King. Later on in the seventeenth century, the Perrault version with the pumpkin and Fairy Godmother reflects the fashions of the court of Louis XIV in France. Patriarchal attitudes are portrayed, Zipes maintains, by emphasising Cinderella's helplessness and her industrious nature as a housekeeper. He points out that the version presented by the Brothers Grimm in their 1812 collection shows the matrilineal strand again. This is characterised by the benign influence of Cinderella's late mother working via the tree and the dove. He suggests that here again the young woman is simply domesticated in order to become worthy of a King. He cites industriousness, self-denial and obedience as qualities of the middle class Protestant ethic. However, as I see it, the Germanic Cinderella is neither helpless nor inactive; and, as Robert Bly points out, there is an essential value in the Journey to the Ashes.

European variants include Ashenputtel (a male example), Rashin Coatie, Mossy Coat and Katie Woodencloak.

Maria Tatar, in 'The Classic Fairy Tales' a collection edited by her, writes of Cinderella, referring to the varying versions: 'She is sometimes cruel and vindictive, at other times compassionate and kind.' 'She can appear genteel and self-effacing in one story, clever and enterprising in another, coy and manipula-tive in a third.' Over time 'the shrewd, resourceful heroine of folktales from earlier centuries has been supplanted by a 'pas-sive princess' waiting for Prince Charming to rescue her. Disney's Cinderella is no match for some of her folkloric ancestors, who refuse to stay at home suffering in silence and who become adept at engineering their own rescues.'

Amongst the many variants, plots either involve 'the anx-ious jealousy of biological and stepmothers', or are 'fueled by the sexual desire of fathers, whose unseemly behaviour drives their daughters from home.'

Typical of this second kind is the tale of the King whose wife dies; he has her wedding ring and makes a vow to marry only that woman whose finger the ring fits. After much searching, his own daughter is found to be the only one whom the ring fits. She then has to get away from him. This group of tales is less familiar to the modern reader. Commentators suggest that they have been in effect suppressed over time because of difficulties and taboos in our society that surround this theme. (This aspect is reflected particularly in Case 10. 'After my mother left my fa-ther put me on a pedestal, he even called me my mother's name.') Another typical example of this type is the tale of Catskin.

Maria Tatar describes these two main types: A) 'an unbear-able family situation is produced by the father's remarriage.' The new wife treats her stepdaughter badly; B) the 'erotic persecu-tion of the daughter by her father' - in these the 'stepmothers and her daughters tend to vanish from the central arena of ac-tion. A + B together combine to produce an intrigue correspond-ing to the oedipal fantasies of girls.' 'Psychoanalitic criticism has indeed seen' the tales 'as enactments of oedipal desires', with each one 'suppressing one component (love for the father or ha-tred of the mother) of the oedipal plot.'

'It is important to bear in mind that the passive or ab-sent father was, even a century ago, not the rule in fairy tales.' 'Cinderella and her cousins were once almost as likely to flee the household because of their father's perverse erotic attachment to them or because of his insistence on a verbal declaration of love, as they were to be banished to the hearth and degraded to domestic servitude by an ill-tempered stepmother.'

In the Catskin type mothers set conditions for the father's

remarriage after their death, which lead him to the daughter as the perfect fit for the ring, or as the only woman equal to the mother in beauty and goodness. These tales include a critique of paternal authority and an endorsement of filial disobedience.

Marian Roalfe observes (in the 1890's) that 'the Catskin stories, originally brilliant and widespread have been reduced to a state of temporary obscurity and eclipse.' Incestuous themes – culturally a sensitive area, at that time and since.

Maria Tatar continues: 'What these stories demonstrate . . . is the way in which the path to happy heterosexual union depends on a successful transfer of filial love from a father to a 'prince,' from a false 'perfect fit' to a true 'perfect fit.'

The male Cinderella type stories.

Maria Tatar again: 'These tales neutralize the persecutions of a wicked stepmother with the sustenance, nurturing, and rescue provided by an animal that is clearly identified with the dead mother.' 'That male Cinderellas have disappeared from our own cultural horizon challenges us to understand exactly what it was that once allowed both girls and boys to participate in the developmental trajectory outlined in the tale.'

Final thoughts.

That this type of tale ends with the the Prince presenting the shoe or ring (both female symbolically) to find the perfect fit with the potential Princess's foot or finger (male symbolically) suggests to me that the tales (and, in some instances, Plastic wrap as a medicine) relate to the search for an equal and pefectly fitting match between the male-female aspects *within* a person – an inner marriage. This inner match may then find its evident manifestation in a flourishing intimate relationship with the 'perfect' partner.

I think it may be valid and useful to extend these considerations, as it were backwards to the time of conception. For each of us coming in, this was the moment in time and place when we first 'experienced' the succesful meeting and matching of these male and female energies and qualities. That particular ovum and sperm met. Precisely.

Imagine the place at the base of an oak tree where the ready acorn was 'received' by the ready soil. The tree grows up, down and out from that seeding time and place.

We all arise from (or sit on) the energy of our conception. Like a tree, we grow from, and in continuing connection to that moment of successful fertilisation. As I understand it, we 'come in' to an exact and fitting match: of male-female aspects, and that this is the case whatever the outer circumstances of the conception might be. Nature doing its thing. When the flower opens, the bees show up. I associate this, in the Plastic proving and cases, with the theme of naturalness developing in various ways: the image of flowering, or of a plant enabled to grow when it had been covered or squashed before.

As life unfolds from the point of conception, this lively and equal match of energies may become disturbed and unequal, sooner or later. This could come about, for example, if the father was absent in any way, or if the mother became distant emotionally. The 'envelope' of energies in which the child develops will be more or less well-balanced in these respects. As the child grows in its world, its own inner male-female aspect will be affected by outer influences, most obviously by the parents' own balance in these respects, but also by the society and its tendencies. This growth pattern may show as a loss of naturalness, or natural ease within the person.

In some instances, this loss may find its remedy in Plastic wrap. (Remember that plastics in the food chain probably influence sexual hormones.)

I have witnessed such benefits as recorded in the cases. It is a joy to see the light of natural aliveness shining again.

Bibliography

*345 Variants of the Cinderella Story. Marian Rolfe Cox. 1893. British Library.
*The Classic Fairy Tales. Maria Tatar (editor). W.W. Norton + Co. Inc. 1999.
*The Brothers Grimm. Jack Zipes. Palgrave Macmillan. 2002.
*Grimms Fairy Tales. Routledge and Kegan Paul. 1975.
*The Chinese Cinderella Story. Arthur Waley. The Journal Folklore No.58. 1947. British Library.
*Tree Medicine, Tree Magic. Ellen Evert Hopman. 1991.
*The Living Wisdom of Trees. Fred Hageneder. Duncan Baird Publishers. 2005.
*The Continuum Encyclopaedia of Symbols. Udo Becker. New York. 2005 reprint.
*English Fairy Tales. Joseph Jacobs. 1890
*Iron John. Robert Bly. 1990

CHAPTER TEN

The Plastic Era

Greek: Plastikos = fit for moulding, plastos = moulded.

Materials modified or invented for use identify historical periods - the Stone Age, the Iron Age etc. In that sense we are, since the 1950's, in the Plastic Age. Our many plastic products have particular and diverse uses, and remarkable benefits. These are evident and well established, and there will be more to come. However, by now, we have become aware of the downside - questions of toxicity and issues of disposal.

An inherent and, as far as I know, general feature of plastics is that they take ages to biodegrade. The bio-team of air, water, worms, insects, moulds etc. cannot easily do the job for us. For the same reason plastics once formed are difficult to reform or recycle.

We chose cling film for this proving as an example of plastic. The provers experienced their symptoms. For some there were profound and lasting changes. Their responses suggest 'resonance' with the remedy, and indicate a connection with experiences earlier in their lives.

Plastic wrap becomes a serviceable medicine and it has 'turned up' when and where it is needed. (In a similar way Amazon tribes will know and find their necessary medicines in their immediate environment.) By way of the proving and the cases we have come to understand something of the scope and territory of this new medicine - a medicine of our time. Some features seem to reflect the life-style, the spirit of this time: the zeitgeist of the Plastic Era. I reckon that some of the states of being and situations described in the cases and proving are 'symptoms' of Western civilised life during this period.

Cling film is a substance of our time. It now provides a timely medicine. Can we now begin to sense and appreciate connections between the original substance and the Materia Medica?

Neither of the following two numbered sections is intended to be exact or complete, so you may well think to make additions or changes. However, comparing the two sections may provide some pointers to the relationship that exists between the material and its Materia Medica.

A signature is unique to a person. Likewise Plastic wrap has its unique 'signature'.

1/ Plastic and plastic wrap as substances.

Plastic. That which can take on many forms. Malleable. Mouldable. Pliable. Unyielding. Impermeable to water or air. Will burn but toxic. Slow to change, slow to biodegrade. Nevertheless volatile. Toxic fume smell of synthetics, carpets and fabrics, and other non food contact plastics. Gets up your nose. Moves. Gets into food and drink? Itself inedible. Hard. Lightweight. Strong. Brittle. Bright and highly coloured. Barbie dolls and Action man – icons of the Plastic Age. Easy to clean. Surface. Uniform, flat appearance. Convenience. The short term advantages. Cheap to produce. Often not prized or valued. Disposable. Throw it away. In sea water it's everywhere, every cubic centimetre. Petroleum derived chemicals in our drinking water? In rainwater?

Product of oil. Oil hardened. Transformed from dirty, fluid, oozing oil to become moulded hard or soft, ultra-clean, even transparent.

Oil - from slow decay of ancient life's debris, underground away from the air and the light of day. Oil doesn't mix with water.

As wrap. Like a skin. Impermeable divider/barrier. Keeps foods from air, from 'natural' progression, from entropy, from decay. Inside the plastic wrap: moisture kept in, food kept 'fresh.' Effects – cannot 'breathe'. Cheese 'sweats'.

Appearance. Transparent. Food looks shiny. Entirely visible but sealed in a protective (defensive) layer.

Water: used in the substance mix and making; once made, the film is a barrier to water.

Wrap. Envelop. Contain. Smother? Restrain. Holding in. Warm. Protect. Defend. Separate. Enclose. Seal off. Define. Embrace closely.

2/ Plastic wrap as medicine.

As discovered from the proving and clinical use.

Relationships issues. Open-ness. Closed. Needing to express. Panic and overwhelm. Feels trapped. Have to get out. Cautious. Self-doubt. Separate. Cannot be at ease in public places, typically at the supermarket! Withdrawn. No joy. Not alive. Dulled.
States of mind and emotions.
About life : Absence of joy and motivation. Loss of natural love of life. Loss of facial colour and brightness about the person. Dulled, wan appearance. Washed out look. Loss (in a ten year old girl) of the natural verve and vitality that had been so striking in her as a young child. Not grounded. Separate from 'natural' world.
In relation to others : Appearance. Acutely self-conscious, when being seen by others. Does not like his/her body, as it is. Thinks he/she is not attractive – au naturel. Has to put on a front, uses make-up and/or behaviour as a mask. "You know, it's not about feeling cool, it's about looking cool." (I heard this recently passing two teenage boys in the street. It seemed to sum up this aspect nicely!) Wanting to attract attention at the same time as not feeling attractive, and acutely anxious about this. Vivacity, chatty and surface euphoria with a compulsive need to be at the centre of attention, in a childish way.
Procrastinates.
In family or other close relationships : Feelings of inadequacy and being judged, for aspects of appearance as well as capabilities. Or, *in intimate relationships*, scared at the moments of connection and joining, 'Feeling I'm caught or losing something - I want to get out of it as quickly as possible.'

In the proving and cases the medicine seems to release a true, simply natural attractiveness, comparable with changes that take place when a woman is ovulating.
In relation to family demands : A mother, feeling overwhelmed, and with a desire to escape from the pressure of her everyday situation.
In the home : Over-concerned about domestic cleanliness and order.

Other features:

Modalities. > open air; > expressing withheld thoughts and feelings.

Skin. Rough, chapped skin < cold weather. Fingernails flaking.

Sensitive to noise and smells. Affected by the volatile smells of synthetic fabrics, e.g. carpets, or upholstery in buses, or by house paints.

Throat. Tension. Fear of choking. Difficulty swallowing. Need to express, to sing. Breathless from exertion.

Dreams : of difficulties, of being pursued, of fights, of escape; of water.

In relation to water : The sacral chakra. Dreams of water. Sensations as if feet are in warm/cold water. Thirstless or thirsty. Drunk sensation after drinking water.

In relation to alcohol : Provers noted an increased effect from even small quantities of alcohol.

Abdomen. Unsettled, 'butterflies' feeling. Panic states.

Male. Less Preoccupied with sexual fantasies. For a man the thought could be "Am I masculine enough to attract a woman?" Macho stance hides this?

Female. As a hormonal remedy, periods and PMT affected. Enjoying being a woman; content, even pleased with her body and 'looks' as is.

Concluding thoughts.

For a while now, I have thought of Princess Diana's life as an example of the themes of the remedy, as well as showing some resonance with the Cinderella archetype. Reading Andrew Morton's biographical books I am fully confirmed in my hunch. Ingredients: Mother absent in her childhood; her own upset she wasn't a boy (to continue the family name), difficult relationship with step-mother and a later reconciliation, thought by the step-mum not to be as beautiful as her two elder sisters, self-doubt, low self-esteem, not accepting her body 'as it is,' dependent for confidence in public on just the right hair cut etc., self-harming, bulimia, difficulties in relationships, feeling trapped and desperate to escape, a love of swimming and diving (brilliant at that as a teenager apparently), finding support from the religious/spiritual dimension. It is curious to note that she died the year that the remedy was made up.

Clinical experience continues to bring consolidation and proof of the proving, doubtless with more to come. As homoeopaths witnessing uses for this remedy, we have begun to associate it with certain trends of recent years – a preoccupation with appearance, clothes, make-up, gloss; a contemporary ideal of perfect looks which can lock into low self-esteem; the need for the new, gadgets, the throw away society; also with broken families which can lead to divided or erratic parenting, step-parent/child difficulties, also the loss or absence of one parent.

My aim with this book has been to make the information accessible to the interested reader as well as for ready use by homoeopaths. It is surprising what we have learnt when you think of the original substance. Perhaps we can claim to demonstrate, with this detailed evidence from the proving and subsequent cases, ways in which we as individuals and in society are being affected during this our Plastic Age. How that works is quite mysterious. Some of us, evidently, are more affected than others. I believe there an accumulative and unbalancing effect on both intimate and social relationships.

The remedy can serve to re-establish natural ease in both these areas. It can bring rich benefits to individuals, to relationships and to the social fabric.

Goethe - Wonder is the beginning of understanding.

Chemist in the plastics industry – "I wonder what substance we will create if we mix these ingredients?"
Homoeopath – "I wonder what will happen if we make a medicine from cling film and then do a proving?"
All of us - wonder at the connection between substance and its medicinal territory!

Full of wonder.

Awesome.

We have discovered mediciinal properties in Plastic wrap. The work has gone on long enough now, and begins to bear fruit. We have used a good long rope, intending to get to the bottom of the matter. It is a deep well, this particular nipple of Mother Earth. May you be refreshed by what you have found here. Let it be known to others who may need it. *Midsummer 2009*

Bibliography

The Dynamics and Methodology of Homoeopathic Provings. Jeremy Sherr. 1994.

Homeopathic Medical Repertory. Robin Murphy. Second Edition 2003.

The Companion to Homoeopathy. Colin Griffith. Watkins 2005.

The New Materia Medica. Colin Griffith. Watkins 2007.

Prometheus. The Journal of the Guild of Homoeopaths No 1 1994 & No 11 December 1999.

Meditative Provings. Madeleine Evans. The Rose Press 2000.

The Elements of the Chakras. Naomi Ozaniec. Clement Books. 1996.

Homoeopathy and Minerals. Jan Scholten. 1993.

Diana. Her True Story. Andrew Morton. London. O'Mara. 1992.

Diana in Pursuit of Love. Andrew Morton. London. O'Mara. 2004.

Of interest –
The film Plastic Planet. Germany. September 2009.
http://www.plastic-planet.at

Recent research results –
Endocrine disruptors in bottled mineral water. Total estrogenic burden and migration from plastic bottles. Martin Wagner and Jorg Oehlmann. Published on line March 2009.
www.springerlink.com
Online pdf see:
www.springerlink.com/content/515wg76276q18115/fulltext.pdf

APPENDIX

The Clinging Film

Plastic Wrap: Invention, Chemistry & Manufacture.

Plastic is the general common term for a wide range of synthetic or semi-synthetic organic amorphous solid materials suitable for the manufacture of industrial products. Plastics are typically polymers of high molecular weight, and may contain other substances to improve performance and/or reduce costs.

The word derives from the Greek 'plastikos' meaning fit for moulding, and 'plastos' meaning moulded. It refers to their malleability, or plasticity during manufacture, that allows them to be cast, pressed, or extruded into an enormous variety of shapes — such as films, fibres, plates, tubes, bottles, boxes, and much more.

The invention of plastic cling wrap

As with many discoveries, Plastic wrap's history is built on a lab error and serendipity. It was invented in 1953 by a scientist who was trying to make a hard plastic cover for his car; his experiment was unsuccessful but he then realised the usefulness of the plastic wrap which he happened to create instead. The original cling wrap material was known as 'Saran' wrap, the commercial name for polyvinylidene chloride (PVdCl). The material was given approval for direct dry food contact and for paperboard coating for contact with fatty and aqueous foods.

In Australia, an early cling wrap material was polyethylene with a 'stickifier' in the form of edible gum. This product was introduced under the brand name 'Glad' in 1966.

Chemistry & Manufacture

My last, and most recent piece of research was to find out about the constituents of a typical plastic wrap, and how it is put together in a factory. I was greatly assisted in this by Jason

199

Leadbitter, an expert in plastics chemistry. SD.

To make Plastic wrap there are four fundamental ingredients as well as other minor ingredients. I indicate the principle reason for their inclusion:

1 PVC Resin - basic plastic ingredient.

2 Plasticisers – polymeric and monomeric – create flexibility and the cling effect.

3 Calcium Zinc Stearate – acts as thermal stabiliser thereby protecting the PVC during manufacture.

4 Epoxidised Soya Bean Oil – acts both as secondary plasticiser as well as a co-stabiliser.

The making of each of these requires chemical laboratory processes, starting with various source substances.

An asterisk* will lead you to an explanation, also highlighted by italics.

The Chemistry and Manufacuture of Poly Vinyl Chloride (PVC) Resin.

Polyvinyl chloride is a synthetic *polymer** produced by polymerization of the *monomer** vinyl chloride. Since a significant proportion of its mass is chlorine, creating a given mass of PVC requires less petroleum than many other polymers, and thereby provides a competitively cost effective product. It is made up of 43% *hydrocarbon**, and 57% chloride components.

A hydrocarbon is a chemical compound of hydrogen and carbon. The hydrocarbon used for PVC comes from either oil derivatives, in a liquid form or from a gas form. Both sources are converted to the hydrocarbon gas known as ethene, more commonly known within the industry as *ethylene**, with the formula C_2H_4. Because it contains a carbon-carbon double bond, ethylene is called an unsaturated hydrocarbon or an alkene. It is the simplest alkene.

In plants, naturally occurring ethylene acts physiologically as a hormone. It exists as a gas and acts at trace levels throughout the life of the plant by stimulating or regulating the ripening of fruit, the opening of flowers, and the shedding of leaves. Tomatoes, bananas and apples will ripen faster in the presence of ethylene. Bananas placed next to other fruits will produce enough ethylene to cause accelerated fruit ripening. Ethylene will shorten the shelf life of cut flowers and potted plants by accelerating the 'aging' process.

A monomer (from the Greek 'mono' one and 'meros' part) is a small molecule that may become chemically bonded to other monomers to form a polymer.

Examples of synthetic monomers are hydrocarbons such as the alkene and arene series. Hydrocarbon monomers such as phenylethene and ethelyne form polymers used as plastics.

The most common natural monomer is glucose, which is linked by glycosidic bonds into polymers such as cellulose and starch, and is over 33% of the weight of all plant matter. Amino acids are natural monomers, and polymerize to form proteins. Nucleotides, monomers found in the cell nucleus, polymerize to form nucleic acids - most famously, DNA and RNA.

A polymer (from the Greek 'polis' much, many and 'meros' part) is a large molecule composed of repeating structural units, typically connected by covalent chemical bonds. While polymer in popular usage suggests plastic, the term actually refers to a large class of natural and synthetic materials with a variety of properties.

Due to the extraordinary range of properties accessible in polymeric materials, they play an essential and ubiquitous role in everyday life, - from plastics and elastomers on the one hand to natural biopolymers such as DNA and proteins that play crucial roles in biological processes.

Synthetic polymers. A simple example is polyethylene, whose repeating unit is based on the ethylene monomer. Most commonly, as in this example, the continuously linked backbone of a polymer consists mainly of carbon atoms.

The list of synthetic polymers includes synthetic rubber, Bakelite, neoprene, nylon, PVC, polystyrene, polypropylene, polyethylene, polyacrylonitrile, PVB, silicone, and many more.

Natural polymeric materials such as shellac, amber, and natural rubber have been in use for centuries. Proteins and nucleic acids are natural polymers. A variety of other natural polymers exist, such as cellulose, which is the main constituent of *wood and paper.*

In PVC manufacture the 57% Chloride component - Ethylene dichloride (EDC) is an *organochloride**

An organochloride, organochlorine, chlorocarbon, or chlorinated solvent is an organic compound containing at least one covalently bonded chlorine atom. Their wide structural variety and divergent chemical properties lead to a broad range of applications.

It is prepared by reacting ethylene and chlorine. The chlorine is produced from Sodium Chloride, common salt. The production of the monomer vinyl chloride from ethylene dichloride (EDC) consists of a series of well-defined steps. In the presence of iron (III) chloride as a catalyst, these compounds react *exothermically**

An exothermic reaction is a chemical reaction that is accompanied by the release of heat. In other words, the energy needed for the reaction to occur is less than the total energy released. As a result of this, extra energy is released, in this case in the form of heat.

Here is the chemical formula for this reaction:

$CH_2=CH_2 + Cl_2\_ClCH_2CH_2Cl$

When heated to 500 °C at 15–30 atmospheres pressure, EDC decomposes to produce vinyl chloride and HCl.

$ClCH_2CH_2Cl\_CH_2=CHCl + HCl$

To deal with the release of heat a propylene refrigerant may be used to chill the outlet stream before it goes into to a series of distillation towers. Pure HCl arises from the top of the last distillation tower, and vinyl chloride comes out of the bottom. The recycled HCl is used to produce more EDC.

Vinyl chloride is the organic compound with the formula $CH_2:CHCl$. At room temperature, vinyl chloride is a gas with a sickly sweet odor that is easily condensed. It is highly toxic and therefore its use by the industry is strictly controlled.

Polyvinyl chloride is produced by polymerization of the vinyl chloride monomer (VCM).

By far the most widely used production process is suspension polymerization. In this process, VCM and water are introduced into the polymerization reactor and a polymerization initiator, along with other chemical additives, are added as catalysts to initiate the polymerization reaction. The contents of the reaction vessel are continually mixed to maintain the suspension and ensure a uniform particle size of the PVC resin. The reaction is exothermic, and thus requires a cooling mechanism to maintain the reactor contents at the appropriate temperature. As the volumes also contract during the reaction (PVC is denser than VCM), water is continually added to the mixture to maintain the suspension.

Once the reaction has run its course, the resulting PVC slurry is degassed and stripped of any residual VCM (which is recycled into the next batch) then passed though a centrifuge to remove most of the excess water. The slurry is then dried further in a hot air bed and the resulting powder sieved before storage or pelletization. The powder looks like fine white salt but is insoluble. In normal operations, the resulting PVC has a VCM content of less than 1 part per million thereby making it suitable for use in food contact applications.

In this way the liquid gas monomer is transformed into a solid by the joining up of atoms, producing a polymer. The reaction time takes a few hours.

The product of the polymerization process is called unmodified PVC. It is inert and benign in respect of skin contact.

As a matter of interest there are a number of people with allergies to latex, and invariably PVC disposable gloves rather than latex are used in hospitals; this could be either for the medical professional or the person who is being operated on.

Before PVC can be made into finished products, it almost always requires conversion into a compound by the incorporation of additives. In the case of cling film these would be a plasticiser, a stabiliser and a plasticiser/co-stabiliser.

If a grain of the powder of PVC is examined under an electron microscope it can be seen to be full of holes. i.e. it is porous. These holes soak in the plasticiser, which is part of the next stage in the production of cling film. From here on there are no more chemical reactions.

So we now bring together the ingredients, as listed on page 200.

1 **PVC resin.**

+

2 **Monomeric and polymeric plasticisers.**

A typical monomeric plasticiser used in the preparation of cling film is Di(2-ethylhexyl) adipate, or DEHA. DEHA is an *ester** of *2-ethylhexanol** and *adipic acid.** Its chemical formula is $C_{22}H_{42}O_4$. It is runny, slightly thicker than water. Adipic acid, as used here, is petroleum oil derived.

An acid + an alcohol produces an ester + water.

Adipic acid is the organic compound with the formula $(CH_2)_4(CO_2H)_2$. From the industrial perspective, it is the most important dicarboxylic acid: about 2.5 billion kilograms of this white crystalline powder are produced annually, mainly as a precursor for the production of nylon. Adipic acid otherwise rarely occurs in nature. Historically, adipic acid was prepared from various fats using oxidation. Currently adipic acid is produced from a mixture of cyclohexanol and cyclohexanone called "KA oil", the abbreviation of "ketone-alcohol oil." The KA oil is oxidized with nitric acid to give adipic acid, via a multistep pathway.

+

2-Ethylhexanol (2-EH), or isooctanol, is a fatty alcohol derived from an organic compound used in the manufacture of a variety of products. It is a branched, eight-carbon alcohol. It is a clear, colourless liquid that is nearly insoluble in water, but well soluble in most organic solvents.

The polymeric plasticiser is a much more viscous liquid rather like thick honey. A typical example is a polymeric adipate such as those manufactured from polyesters of adipic acid and propanediols and/or polypropylene glycol, end capped with acetic acid or fatty acids or n-octanol and/or n-decanol.

Proportions of monomeric and polymeric plasticizers, and health concerns.

A typical cling film will comprise a specific ratio of monomeric and polymeric plasticisers; the reason being that monomeric plasticisers have a chemical attraction to fatty foods like cheese and hence can migrate away from the packaging and into the foodstuff itself. So, in recent years there has been an increase in the proportion of polymeric plasticiser used. This has bigger molecules and so the rate of migration is significantly lower. This appears to have been the industry's considered response to public concern about possibility of toxicity resulting from the migration of DEHA, the most common monomeric plasticiser used in cling film.

Suspicion of toxicity versus scientific knowledge.

In rodent studies, during which DEHA was administered at very high doses – many, many times higher than would ever be experienced by humans during everyday use of cling film – there has been evidence of liver cancer. However, the significant species differences that exist between the ways in which a human liver and a rodent liver respond to DEHA means that carcinogenicity in humans from DEHA exposure is extremely unlikely.

There is no validated scientific evidence to suggest that DEHA is an endocrine disrupter.

There is no evidence that DEHA causes human reproductive problems. It is true that DEHA, at high dose levels, has been shown to cause reproductive effects in rats and mice. However, the relevance of these findings to humans is limited due to the dose level being far in excess of human exposure and the fact that primates appear to be resistant to the reproductive effects seen in rodents.

Yet for all its versatility and obvious benefits, there has been media speculation about its safety. Whatever material is chosen for packaging food there is always some transfer from the constituents of the package to foodstuffs. A considerable amount of experimental work has been carried out to determine the migration from plasticised PVC into food.

In tests conducted in the UK and more recently in France, Germany, and the Netherlands, it was shown that the average DEHA intake was six to twenty times below the limits proposed by the EC Scientific Committee for Food which already have large margins of safety built in.

+

3 **Calcium Zinc Stearate. CZS.** This is added to thermally protect the PVC composition during the heater mixing and transforming of the PVC compound into the final film, a process which requires relatively high temperatures on various rollers (calendering) – under pressure. Without this additive the PVC would degrade.

CZS is made from stearic acid combined with the elements calcium and zinc. The stearic acid used to come from the fat of herded cattle, but since concerns over BSE, most companies now use stearic acid derived from vegetable oil, rapeseed for example, as a source.

+

4 **Epoxidised soya oil**. This additive has a duel function both serving as a secondary stabiliser and as an additional plasticiser within the product. Its manufacturing process relies on the addition of epoxy groups to Soya bean oil. It is epoxidised (made more sticky) with CH_2CH_2O. The epoxy group provides the necessary compatibility with the polymer.

My chemist advisor suggested to me that if any alterative effects could be attributed to cling film then we should not rule out potential phyto-oestrogenic effects of the soya bean constituent of the wrap. SD

The final stage.

In order to manufacture cling film the above ingredients would first be mixed in a high speed mixer which generates heat as well as allowing the plasticisers to be absorbed by the PVC resin with good dispersion of the stabilizer. Once the mixing has achieved an acceptable level of dispersion the film is manufactured by the process known as calendering which produces extremely thin sheets at very high speeds through a series of rollers which ultimately determine the required thickness. Water is used to keep the rollers clear.

Connections with contemporary homoeopathic understanding.

Homoeopaths are familiar with the therapeutic scope and Materia Medica of other Chloride remedies. These include the medicine made from salt, Sodium Chloride (Latin name Natrum muriaticum), as well as Potassium, Magnesium and Calcium Chlorides.

Jan Scholten, a Dutch homoeopath draws attention to five features as recurrent Materia Medica themes of remedies made from other Chlorides:

Self-pity   Care and nurturing

Mother (meaning issues of mothering or
relationship with the mother)

(Need for) attention and Self-awareness

Jan Scholten - Homoeopathy and Minerals 1993

Common salt, as we have seen is the source ingredient for the Chlorine that goes into the making of Ethylene di-chloride. This in turn is a constituent of PVC and then Plastic wrap. Perhaps this is why we see these themes showing up in the proving and cases.

Equally I propose that the ethylene component of the substance is reflected in the instances of hormonal changes and maturation – ripening.

POSTSCRIPT

Woman, aged 25. Summer Of 2009.

The Plastic remedy came to me last year at a time of intense discovery in my life - the transitionary period between childhood and womanhood. Fed up with feeling small, diminished, inadequate and full of rage towards the world, my self, my mother and society, I was pretty desperate to take control and release old patterns that I could so clearly see were holding me back, and to whose beat I no longer wanted to dance. The remedy came with me on my first solo trip to Asia, and it was invaluable at widening my perspective and softening my fear, assisting me in moving through these feelings instead of what I had been doing for years - battling, suffering, and taking it out primarily on myself and my body. I now feel more grounded, more spacious, more empowered, safer, more myself, than ever before, and deeply appreciate the support that the remedy gives me as I continue to grow and experience.